Introduction to Approaches in Music Therapy

Second Edition

Introduction to Approaches in Music Therapy

Second Edition

೪

Edited by

Alice-Ann Darrow

American Music Therapy Association, Inc.

The American Music Therapy Association is a non-profit association dedicated to increasing access to quality music therapy services for individuals with disabilities or illnesses or for those who are interested in personal growth and wellness. The mission of the American Music Therapy Association is to advance public awareness of the benefits of music therapy and increase access to quality music therapy services in a rapidly changing world. AMTA provides extensive educational and research information about the music therapy profession. Referrals for qualified music therapists are also provided to consumers and parents. AMTA holds an annual conference every autumn and its seven regions hold conferences every spring.

For up-to-date information, please access the AMTA website at www.musictherapy.org

ISBN: 978-1-884914-21-8

Editor: **Alice-Ann Darrow, PhD, MT-BC**
Florida State University
Tallahassee, Florida

Copyright Information: **© by American Music Therapy Association, Inc. 2008**
8455 Colesville Road, Suite 1000
Silver Spring, MD 20910 USA
www.musictherapy.org
info@musictherapy.org

Technical Assistance: **Wordsetters**
Kalamazoo, Michigan

Cover Design: **Tawna Grasty, Grass T Design**

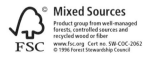

Printed in the United States of America

Contents

Preface vii

Acknowledgments ix

1   What's in a Name? An Introduction to Approaches
    in Music Therapy... 1

Section One: Approaches Adapted From Music Education 9

2   The Orff Approach to Music Therapy 11

3   The Dalcroze Approach to Music Therapy 25

4   The Kodály Approach to Music Therapy..................................... 37

Section Two: Psychotherapeutic Approaches to Music Therapy 47

5   The Bonny Method of Guided Imagery and Music....................... 49

6   Nordoff-Robbins Music Therapy 61

7   Psychodynamic Approach to Music Therapy 79

8   Behavioral Approach to Music Therapy..................................... 105

Section Three: Medical Approaches to Music Therapy 129

9   Music Therapy in Wellness 131

10 Neurologic Music Therapy 153

11 The Biomedical Theory of Music Therapy 173

Preface

Before joining the faculty at Florida State University in the fall of 2003, I had the good fortune to spend the first 20 years of my career at The University of Kansas. One of the graduate courses I taught while at KU was the Philosophy and Theory of Music Therapy. In this course, we had an exceptional group of graduate students who expressed interest in researching the wide range of approaches to music therapy. Many of these students had studied at other universities and were already familiar with many of the approaches included in this book. These students became the leaders of organized research and writing teams. I was also fortunate to have competent and cooperative colleagues at The University of Kansas who agreed to collaborate with the students on their research and writing efforts. Thus began the cooperative projects that resulted in *Introduction to Approaches in Music Therapy*.

In preparing the first edition, I felt it was imperative, as editor, to get experts in each of the approaches to review the chapters. Based on their reviews, chapters were revised. In an effort to further ensure the integrity of the approach descriptions, I invited guest authors to complete chapters that required special expertise. I am grateful and indebted to the reviewers and guest authors for making the first edition a sincere effort at introducing the many different approaches to music therapy. Because the chapters in the first edition were thoroughly appraised by the reviewers, and later by users of the text, reviewers were not employed for the second edition. However, in order to maintain the integrity of the approach descriptions, guest authors used in the first edition were asked to be the first authors of their chapters, and with one exception, these individuals were responsible for all revisions in the second edition. The one exception was Chapter 7, The Psychodynamic Approach to Music Therapy, for which Connie Isenberg and Francis Smith Goldberg were responsible for authoring this chapter for the second edition. A substantial change in the second edition is the inclusion of an introductory chapter, and deletion of a chapter, Kindermusik and Music Therapy. This chapter was deleted because it is no longer a part of common practice in music therapy, and because current research does not support its merit as a form of music therapy practice.

Introduction to Approaches in Music Therapy is written for entering students in music therapy programs, or anyone who wants to know more about music therapy. It is also written with the hopes that we, as professionals, can appreciate and become more familiar with approaches that may not be our own and, consequently, take pride in the rich diversity within our profession.

The book is organized into three major sections: Approaches Adapted from Music Education, Psychotherapeutic Approaches to Music Therapy, and Medical Approaches to Music Therapy. These sections also approximate the historical development of the music therapy profession. In the early years of music therapy, many of the techniques used were borrowed and adapted from other related professions. As music therapy clinical practice increased, music therapists developed specialized approaches that were unique to our profession. And while music therapy has a well established place in the history of medicine, it was not until recent years that early practices were organized into specific music therapy approaches.

The organization of chapters is similar. Each chapter begins with an introduction to or overview of a specific approach to music therapy. Also included in each chapter is the history or background of the approach, description of the approach—including philosophical orientation, clinical applications of the approach, related research, summary or conclusions, references, and suggestions for further reading.

I hope that *Introduction to Approaches in Music Therapy* provides readers with the opportunity to increase their knowledge of music therapy, but more importantly, I hope it prompts readers to appreciate the versatility of music and to respect the diversity of approaches that comprise our profession.

Acknowledgments

In editing this book, I was given the opportunity to work with talented graduate students who are all now accomplished professionals in the field, collaborate with colleagues, consult with recognized experts in the profession of music therapy, and communicate regularly with authors whose contributions significantly increased my knowledge of music therapy. I would like to express special appreciation to the reviewers of the first edition of this book for their important contributions to that edition. Their credentials and places of employment are listed below. I would like to give special acknowledgment to Carol Bitcon, a former president of our national association, and to Helen Bonny. In their retirement, they reviewed and provided comments on the chapters "The Orff Approach to Music Therapy" and "The Bonny Method of Guided Imagery and Music."

Authors

Kenneth Aigen, DA, MT-BC
Faculty, The Nordoff-Robbins Center for Music Therapy at New York University, New York, New York
Chapter 6: Nordoff-Robbins Music Therapy

Mike D. Brownell, MME, MT-BC
Private Practice, Ann Arbor, Michigan
Chapter 4: The Kodály Approach to Music Therapy
Chapter 8: Behavioral Approach to Music Therapy

Debra Burns, PhD, MT-BC
Faculty, Indiana University at IUPUI, Indianapolis
Chapter 5: The Bonny Method of Guided Imagery and Music

Alicia A. Clair, PhD, MT-BC
Faculty, University of Kansas, Lawrence
Chapter 10: Neurologic Music Therapy

Cynthia M. Colwell, PhD, MT-BC
Faculty, University of Kansas, Lawrence
Chapter 2: The Orff Approach to Music Therapy

Alice-Ann Darrow, PhD, MT-BC
Faculty, Florida State University, Tallahassee
Chapter 1: What's in a Name? Introduction to Approaches in Music Therapy

Janice M. Dvorkin, PsyD, ACMT
Faculty, University of the Incarnate Word, San Antonio, Texas
Chapter 7: Psychodynamic Approach to Music Therapy

R. J. David Frego, PhD
Faculty, University of Texas at San Antonio
Chapter 3: The Dalcroze Approach to Music Therapy
Chapter 4: The Kodály Approach to Music Therapy

Acknowledgments

Claire Mathern Ghetti, MME, MT-BC
Doctoral Student, University of
Kansas, Lawrence
Chapter 9: Music Therapy in Wellness

Greta Gillmeister, MT-BC
Music Therapy Services of Central
Kentucky, Louisville
*Chapter 2: The Orff Approach to
Music Therapy*
*Chapter 3: The Dalcroze Approach to
Music Therapy*

Frances Smith Goldberg, MA, MT-BC
Retired, California Institute for Integral
Studies, University of California, San
Francisco
Private Practice, Indianapolis, Indiana
*Chapter 7: Psychodynamic Approach to
Music Therapy*

Mika Hama, MME, MT-BC
Doctoral Student, Georgetown
University, Washington, DC
*Chapter 3: The Dalcroze Approach to
Music Therapy*
Chapter 9: Music Therapy in Wellness

Connie Isenberg, PhD, MT-BC
Faculty, University of Québec at
Montréal, Québec, Canada
*Chapter 7: Psychodynamic Approach to
Music Therapy*

Christopher M. Johnson, PhD
Faculty, University of Kansas, Lawrence
*Chapter 8: Behavioral Approach to
Music Therapy*

Cari Kennedy Miller, MME, MT-BC
Private Practice, Fairport, New York
*Chapter 6: Nordoff-Robbins Music
Therapy*

Shin-Hee Kim
Private Practice, Seoul, Korea
*Chapter 8: Behavioral Approach to
Music Therapy*

Youngshin Kim, PhD, MT-BC
Faculty, Sookmyung Women's
University, Seoul, Korea
*Chapter 6: Nordoff-Robbins Music
Therapy*

Eum-Mi [Emily] Kwak, MME, MT-BC
Doctoral Student, Michigan State
University, East Lansing
*Chapter 4: The Kodály Approach to
Music Therapy*
*Chapter 6: Nordoff-Robbins Music
Therapy*

Blythe LaGasse, MME, MT-BC
Doctoral Student, University of Kansas,
Lawrence
Chapter 10: Neurologic Music Therapy

Robin E. Liston, PhD
Faculty, Baker University, Baldwin,
Kansas
*Chapter 3: The Dalcroze Approach to
Music Therapy*

Varvara Pasiali, MME, MT-BC
Doctoral Student, Michigan State
University, East Lansing
*Chapter 6: Nordoff-Robbins Music
Therapy*
Chapter 10: Neurologic Music Therapy

Carol Achey Pehotsky, MME, MT-BC
The Cleveland Clinic Foundation,
Cleveland, Ohio
*Chapter 2: The Orff Approach to Music
Therapy*

Amanda M. Rayburn, MME, MT-BC
Austin Independent School District,
    Austin, Texas
*Chapter 4: The Kodály Approach to
    Music Therapy*

Sheri L. Robb, PhD, MT-BC
Research Associate, Indiana University
    at IUPUI, Indianapolis
*Chapter 8: Behavioral Approach to
    Music Therapy*

Jayne Standley, PhD, MT-BC
Faculty, Florida State University,
    Tallahassee
*Chapter 8: Behavioral Approach to
    Music Therapy*

Daniel B. Tague, MME, MT-BC
Music Therapy Services of Texas,
    Dallas-Fort Worth
*Chapter 6: Nordoff-Robbins Music
    Therapy*

Dale B. Taylor, PhD, MT-BC
Visiting Professor, Augsburg College,
    Minneapolis, Minnesota
Emeritus Faculty, University of
    Wisconsin–Eau Claire
Chapter 11: Biomedical Music Therapy

Jennifer Woolrich, MME
Private Practice, Bartlesville, Oklahoma
*Chapter 2: The Orff Approach to Music
    Therapy*
*Chapter 5: The Bonny Method of Guided
    Imagery and Music*
Chapter 9: Music Therapy and Wellness

Reviewers

Diane Austin, DA, LCAT, ACMT
Private Practice, New York University
    Turtle Bay Music School
*Chapter 7: Psychodynamic Approach to
    Music Therapy*

Carol Bitcon, MA
Retired
*Chapter 2: The Orff Approach to
    Music Therapy*

Helen Bonny, PhD
Private Practice
*Chapter 5: The Bonny Method of
    Guided Imagery and Music*

Alicia Ann Clair, PhD, MT-BC
University of Kansas
Chapter 9: Music Therapy in Wellness

Nancy Ferguson, PhD (deceased)
Formerly at the University of Arizona
*Chapter 2: The Orff Approach to Music
    Therapy*

Clifford K. Madsen, PhD
Florida State University
*Chapter 8: Behavioral Approach to
    Music Therapy*

Clive Robbins, DHL, DMM, MT-BC
The Nordoff-Robbins Center for Music
Therapy at New York University
*Chapter 6: Nordoff-Robbins Music
Therapy*

Michael Thaut, PhD
Colorado State University
Chapter 10: Neurologic Music Therapy

Concetta M. Tomaino, DA, MT-BC
Institute for Music and Neurologic
Function
Music Therapy Services, Beth Abraham
Family of Health Services
Chapter 11: Biomedical Music Therapy

Alan Turry, MA, NRMT, MT-BC
The Nordoff-Robbins Center for Music
Therapy at New York University
*Chapter 6: Nordoff-Robbins Music
Therapy*

Jayne Wenne, MA
Hilliard City Schools, Hilliard, Ohio
*Chapter 3:The Dalcroze Approach to
Music Therapy*
*Chapter 4: The Kodály Approach to
Music Therapy*

Chapter 1

What's in a Name?
An Introduction to Approaches
in Music Therapy

Alice-Ann Darrow

Introduction

As Shakespeare's Juliet asked, "What's in a name?" Does it matter? Apparently, it does. In the field of music therapy, as with other professions, names carry a great deal of meaning—and they are important to understanding the discipline. In determining the most appropriate title for this text, the first authors of the chapters weighed in on the meaning of the terms *approach* and *method* and which term most accurately portrayed the intent of the individual chapters and the text as a whole. Rightfully so, practitioners of all approaches or methodologies are protective of the terms used to describe their practice, and they are mindful of how these terms are interpreted by others. In some cases, the use of these two terms is based on convention, and in other instances, the terms are quite specific to the music therapy practice they describe. In the end, the term *methods* was thought to be too restrictive or specific, and the term *approaches* was deemed inclusive enough for the purposes of this text.

Within various approaches, there are related terms, such as *intervention*, *strategy*, *procedure*, *protocol*, *process*, or *practice*. In the field of music therapy, these terms relate to therapists' interactions with clients. Music therapists who use the various approaches described in this text are likely to interact with their clients quite differently. How then does one determine what is considered to be "best practice" in the field of music therapy? The term *best practice* is generally regarded—as implied by the word *best*—to be a superior or innovative practice that has been shown to bring about the most desirable results for people or for an organization. *Webster's New Millennium™ Dictionary of English* (2008) defines best practice as "a practice which is most appropriate under the circumstances, especially as considered acceptable or regulated in business; a technique or methodology that, through experience and research, has reliably led to a desired or optimum result."

This definition seems workable for the purposes of this text because it allows for *circumstantial differences*. Proponents of any practice must take into account the individuals and/or circumstances involved. Music therapists—like their clients—are individuals who come to the field of music therapy with different backgrounds, experiences, skills, and philosophies. It is unlikely then that the field of music therapy will ever embrace one single approach as "best practice." Much like medicine, where varying approaches to care and various drugs have all been found to effectively treat patients with the same illness or disorder, evidence-based practice in music therapy has also revealed the benefits of multiple approaches. The diversity of approaches in music therapy practice today allows us as therapists to reach a wider population of clients, and to tailor our work to the unique needs and preferences of our clients.

Historical Perspective on Approaches in Music Therapy

A relationship between music and healing has been acknowledged as far back as early civilizations, though data on its effects, even of an anecdotal nature, did not appear in literature until the late 18th century (Davis & Gfeller, 2008; Horden, 2000). A systematic approach to the application of music was not evident until the mid 1940s (Davis & Gfeller, 2008; Rorke, 1996). During these early years of music therapy growth in the United States, much of what was written about music therapy practice was borrowed or generalized from other fields, particularly the fields of psychotherapy and general wellness programs. At the time, psychotherapy was seen as the most accepted form of treatment for persons with psychosocial disorders, and general wellness programs were a part of the postwar efforts to rehabilitate veterans. It was understandable that music therapists aligned themselves with established practices of care. Music was still viewed by many in health fields as primarily an art form.

As the music therapy profession began to grow, therapists began to establish their own approaches to music therapy practice, approaches that were independent of other practices and that were not viewed as ancillary. One could understandably argue that no approach in music therapy is totally independent, that is, without some foundation in medicine, psychology, or other health-related fields. There are, however, proponents of music therapy approaches who view music as the primary health agent in their approach—and not secondary or subordinate to any other type of intervention. Music as the primary or an independent health agent, though, is not what defines an approach in music therapy. Common practice is one way to address the definition of *approach*, but the notion of common practice presents a major fallacy. In common practice, the fact that most people do X is used as "evidence" to support the action or practice. It is a fallacy because the mere fact that most people do something does not make it correct, moral, justified, or reasonable. There is no clear definition for what constitutes an approach in music therapy.

Again, the question arises, "What's in a name?" And again, the answer is . . . names are important. Names are a means of communicating ideas, establishing identities, differentiating between entities, and declaring uniqueness among other entities. Establishing a name for an approach seems to be at least a start at defining it, since names often identify the origin or nature of the music therapy approach. The first named approach in music therapy was Nordoff-Robbins Music Therapy, named after its founders, Paul Nordoff and Clive Robbins. Guided Imagery and Music (GIM) soon followed as the second named approach. In this text, GIM is referred to as

Bonny Method GIM, or BMGIM in honor of its founder, Helen Bonny. Both of these approaches share foundations in the fields of psychology and philosophy, and particularly in the concepts of self-actualization and humanism.

Nordoff and Robbins believed that all individuals have a musical self, and that by awakening that musicality, they can become more self-aware, more open to therapy, and, ultimately, more communicative and responsive. In developing their music therapy approach, Nordoff and Robbins drew upon the thinking of several philosophers, most notably Rudolf Steiner and his concept of anthroposophy, as well as Abraham Maslow's concept of humanism. Inherent in both Nordoff Robbins Music Therapy and BMGIM is a deep respect for the individuality and humanism of all people.

In a presentation at the World Congress of Music Therapy in 1999, Helen Bonny acknowledged that GIM leans heavily on two psychological forces: humanism and transpersonal, although music is at the core of the approach. The uses of music in GIM are viewed as a major difference between the Bonny Method and traditional music therapy (Bonny, 2002). Classical music is chosen from the masters and listened to in a deeply relaxed state of consciousness. The BMGIM is an example of an approach grounded in a field other than music, but with music serving as the primary agent of change and as its identifying feature. Nordoff-Robbins Music Therapy and BMGIM's founding discipline, psychology, has been a parent field to other approaches in music therapy, and thus constitutes one of the major categories of music therapy approaches.

Categorizing Music Therapy Approaches

Approaches to music therapy generally fall under three categories: approaches adapted from music education, psychotherapeutic approaches to music therapy, and medical approaches to music therapy. These categories are related either to the origin or basis of the approach. Some approaches to music therapy are based on a biological or medical model, while others evolved as direct applications of existent educational approaches or other types of therapy.

Approaches Adapted from Music Education. Music educators, psychologists, anthropologists, and others have long known that music has extra musical benefits—benefits that extend beyond the nature of the music itself. As early as 1964, Merriam, an anthropologist, wrote of the emotional, cultural, social, and spiritual influences of music. Some researchers argue that even the study of music has extra musical benefits (Johnson & Memmott, 2006). MENC: The National Association of Music Educators defends music study as beneficial to students beyond the education it provides (MENC, 2007). The organization suggests that benefits conveyed by music education can be grouped into four categories: success in society, success in school and learning, success in developing intelligence, and success in life. It is not surprising then that some of the approaches used in music therapy are rooted in educational practices.

By the early to mid 20th century, European methods and approaches to music teaching were gaining popularity in the United States. Among these approaches were several that American music educators embraced with particular enthusiasm: Dalcroze, Orff, and Kodály (Campbell & Scott-Kassner, 1995; Mark & Gary, 1992). There was good reason for their enthusiasm. Children who were taught using these approaches excelled in singing, as well as reading and creating music. American music educators were eager to use these approaches with their own students.

As increasing numbers of students with disabilities entered public schools, music educators soon found that certain aspects of these European approaches were useful in teaching students with special needs. Students benefited from the movement aspects of the Dalcroze approach, or from the use of visual aids found in the Kodály approach, or from the kinesthetic function of playing large instruments used in the Orff approach. Because many music therapists have backgrounds or degrees in music education, and some have certification in these European approaches, it was not long until they found ways to incorporate Orff, Dalcroze, and Kodály approaches in their music therapy practice.

Psychotherapeutic Approaches to Music Therapy. These approaches involve the treatment of cognitive, emotional, behavioral, or physical disorders through the use of music techniques designed to provide relief of symptoms, or actual changes in persons' physical, emotional, or behavioral states, thus leading to their improved functioning. Although some of these approaches address physical disorders, they are primarily used to address cognitive, emotional, or behavioral therapeutic objectives. These approaches have very different orientations to client interactions and to methods of assessing outcomes; however, their basic therapeutic purposes are the same— and all relate to the well-being of clients. The approaches included in this section are based on several types of psychotherapy: Psychodynamic Therapy, Interpersonal Therapy, Guided Imagery, Behavior Therapy, and Cognitive Therapy (Corsini & Wedding, 2005).

Sigmund Freud made the earliest contributions to the field of psychotherapy with his descriptions of the unconscious, the use of dreams, and his model of the human mind. Freud believed that mental illness was the result of keeping thoughts or memories in the unconscious, and that through treatment—primarily listening to the patient and providing interpretations— these thoughts and memories could be brought to the forefront of the mind and thus decrease negative symptoms. The goals of psychodynamic therapy are a client's self-awareness and understanding of the influence of the past on present behavior. A psychodynamic approach enables the client to examine unresolved conflicts and symptoms that arise from the past.

Guided imagery is an approach that focuses on directed thoughts and suggestions. These directed thoughts or suggestions can guide one toward a more relaxed and focused state. Guided imagery is based on the concept that the body and mind are connected and, thus, by using all of one's senses, the body responds as though what is imagined is real.

The interpersonal therapy, or the humanistic approach, developed by Carl Rogers focuses on interpersonal relationships. This approach is founded on the idea that by improving persons' communication patterns and how they relate to others, they are then better able to function in daily life. Carl Rogers also believed in transmitting warmth and genuine concern from therapist to client as a part of interpersonal therapy.

Behavior therapy is focused on helping an individual understand how changing their behavior can lead to changes in how they are feeling and in their overall functioning. Behavior therapy is a structured approach that carefully measures what the person is doing and then seeks to increase the likelihood of more positive behaviors. Over the years, behavior therapy has included importance on the thoughts and feelings of the person, which is borrowed from cognitive therapy, an approach based on the theory that much of how we feel is determined by what we think. By correcting inaccurate beliefs, a person's perception of events and emotional state can improve. The combination of these two therapies is known as cognitive-behavioral therapy.

Medical Approaches to Music Therapy. The approaches included under this category have the distinction of addressing medical objectives, or are based in the biological sciences. Medical music therapy is used in general hospitals, rehabilitation centers, or any facility where medical procedures are carried out. Music therapy is used to alleviate pain in conjunction with anesthesia or pain medication; elevate patients' mood and counteract depression; promote movement for physical rehabilitation; calm or sedate, often to induce sleep; counteract apprehension or fear; and lessen muscle tension for the purpose of relaxation, including the autonomic nervous system (American Music Therapy Association, 2008).

The notion that music can affect health and promote healing is as least as old as the writings of Aristotle and Plato (Davis & Gfeller, 2008). The 20th century discipline began in earnest after World War II when U.S. veterans returned home to hospitals for rehabilitation. After doctors and nurses noted their informal responses to music, music programs were set up in veterans' hospitals across the country, sometimes for purely recreational purposes, but often for therapeutic purposes. Over the last 50 years, music therapy has gained increasing popularity in the medical communities, and today many medical and rehabilitation facilities offer music therapy as one of their treatment modalities. The medical approaches included in this text are representative of the history of medical music therapy practice.

The idea of preventative approaches to health gained popularity during the 1970s, and, as a result, wellness programs were organized in corporations, schools, and assisted living and nursing facilities. The accepted notion among medical communities that music could not only prevent illnesses, but also contribute to their cure, came later. This acceptance is due in part to writings by various authors explaining the biological foundations of music therapy, and to empirical evidence supporting the relationship between neuroscience and music as therapy. As music therapy professionals, we are indebted to those who have produced and disseminated the research and, by doing so, have promoted the acceptance of music therapy by the medical communities.

Conclusions

Introduction to Approaches in Music Therapy is a celebration of the rich diversity found in the field of music therapy today. Diversity allows for options in care. Just as clients may desire or require different types of care, music therapists may also desire or need to utilize a variety of approaches in order to meet the diverse needs of their clients. However, some approaches may not be feasible for music therapists to employ in practice. These approaches typically require special skills on the part of the therapist. For example, music therapists who use the Nordoff-Robbins approach in their practice need to be proficient at improvising, and those who use the Bonny Method of Guided Imagery and Music must have a broad knowledge of classical music literature.

Some of the approaches described in this text are aligned with certification programs that train professionals on use of the approach. Upon completion of these programs, professionals are allowed to signify their credentials by using specific initials after their names. There are also different levels of certification for some of the approaches. The time required to complete each level varies depending on the approach and those who regulate or administer the certification program. Certification programs are frequently offered at national conferences of the American Music Therapy Association and at sites across the country.

While reading the various chapters, it is likely that one or several approaches will strike a chord with readers. It may be something in the philosophy or research that they can identify with, or the orientation to the approach may relate to their own backgrounds in education, medicine, or psychology. It is likely too that some readers may not agree with the philosophical basis of a particular approach. Diversity of thought is a natural outcome of growth in the music therapy profession. Again, how fortunate we are to have the richness of diversity and acceptable practice alternatives in the field of music therapy today.

We are also fortunate to have proponents of the major approaches who are passionate about their specific approaches and who can write eloquently about them. The transmission of ideas about music therapy is critical to the growth of the profession, and music therapy has experienced considerable growth over the past 50 years. It is likely the field will continue to grow and to diversify over the next 50 years. Who knows what additional approaches the future holds? While *Introduction to Approaches in Music Therapy* is, as its title implies, an introduction, it is a thorough orientation to the breadth and diversity found in music therapy practice today.

References

American Music Therapy Association (AMTA). (2008). *How is music therapy used in hospitals*? Retrieved March 15, 2008, from http://www.musictherapy.org/faqs.html

Bonny, H. (1999, November). *Plenary session: Panel of founders.* World Congress of Music Therapy, Washington, DC.

Bonny, H. (2002). *Music and consciousness: The evolution of guided imagery and music.* Gilsum, NH: Barcelona.

Campbell, P. S., & Scott-Kassner, C. (1995). *Music in childhood: From preschool through the elementary grades.* New York: Schirmer Books.

Corsini, R. J., & Wedding, D. (Eds.). (2005). *Current psychotherapies* (7th ed.). Belmont, CA: Thomson-Brooks/Cole.

Davis, W. B., & Gfeller, K. (2008). Music therapy: An historical perspective. In W. B. Davis, K. E. Gfeller, & M. H. Thaut (Eds.), *Introduction to music therapy: Theory and practice* (3rd ed.). Silver Spring, MD: American Music Therapy Association.

Horden, P. (2000). *Music as medicine: The history of music therapy since antiquity.* London: Ashgate.

Johnson, C. M., & Memmott, J. E. (2006). Examination of relationship between participation in school music programs of differing quality and standardized test results. *Journal of Research in Music Education, 54,* 293–307.

Mark, M. L., & Gary, C. L. (1992). *A history of American music education.* New York: Schirmer Books.

MENC. (2007). *Why music education? Facts and insights on the benefits of music study* [Brochure]. Reston, VA: MENC: National Association of Music Educators.

Merriam, A. P. (1964). *The anthropology of music.* Evanston, IL: Northwestern University.

Rorke, M. A. (1996). Music and the wounded of World War II. *Journal of Music Therapy, 33*, 189–207.

Webster's New Millennium™ Dictionary of English, Preview Edition (v 0.9.7). (2003–2008). Lexico Publishing Group. Retrieved March 16, 2008, from http://dictionary.reference.com/browse/best%20practice

Section One

Approaches Adapted from Music Education

Chapter 2

The Orff Approach to Music Therapy

Cynthia M. Colwell
Carol Achey Pehotsky
Greta Gillmeister
Jennifer Woolrich

History

Carl Orff's Life

Carl Orff was born July 10, 1895, in Munich, Germany. He grew up in a musical environment where, as in typical homes of this time, it was common for the adults to gather and perform music for each other and as an ensemble. While growing up, Orff was exposed to the rich musical culture of Munich, which included opera, concert music, and drama. At age 5, Orff began piano lessons with his mother, followed by formal music training at the Akademie der Tonkunst.

Orff's involvement in the field of music led to his eventual career choice. In 1915, Orff became the musical director of theater works at the Munich Kammerspiele. During this time, he focused his studies of music on Renaissance and early Baroque composers, whose influences are noted in his own works. Orff also served as the director of the Munich Bach Society until 1933 (American Orff-Schulwerk Association [AOSA], 2000; Warner, 1991).

From 1935 to 1942, Orff devoted his life to composing many stage works. Language was the most important element in these works, serving as the creative foundation for the music he composed around it (Carl Orff Foundation, 1999). His most famous work, *Carmina Burana*, premiered in 1937. Additional works include *Der Mond* (The Moon), *Die Kluge* (The Peasant's Wise Daughter), *Antigonae*, *Trionfi*, and *Prometheus*. His final work, *De Temporum Fine Comoedia* (The Comedy About the End of Time), premiered in 1973 at the Salzburg Festival. After dedicating his life to the field of music, Orff passed away on March 19, 1982, at the age of 86 (AOSA, 2000; Warner, 1991).

Orff Schulwerk

In addition to his work as a composer, Orff dedicated much of his life to an approach to music education that focused on learning by doing. The groundwork was laid in the early 1920s when, through his work as music director of the Guntherschule, he focused his attention on elemental music. The second phase, begun in the late 1940s, saw the focus directed at how this approach was music for children by children.

In 1923, Orff met Dorothee Gunther, an innovative dancer who wished to build a school to teach movement, rhythm, and dance. A year later, the Guntherschule was founded in Munich. The education was based on the use of elemental music—a music that integrates the elements of speech, movement, and dance. Orff focused on rhythm as the foundation for elemental music. He used body sounds and gestures to teach rhythm and incorporated improvisation techniques at the center of his instruction (Rudaitis, 1995; Warner, 1991). Much of the focus on elemental music was due to his desire to seek alternatives to Western music and to find a source for a primitive form for experimentation (Frazee & Kreuter, 1987).

Orff used a variety of instruments, but the voice remained the primary instrument, as he considered it the most natural. He gradually added percussive instruments, with an emphasis on drums. The piano was used initially as it was the only pitched instrument available to him. It was replaced in 1926, when the xylophone, or "Kaffernklavier," was introduced to Orff. Karl Maendler, a harpsichord builder, helped Orff design and build barred instruments for the school modeled after an African xylophone. Gunild Keetman, one of Orff's students at the Guntherschule, developed the techniques to play these instruments and established a standard ensemble for them, the instrumentarium. She also incorporated the recorder into this ensemble, and developed specific techniques to use this instrument in Orff Schulwerk (Warner, 1991).

By 1926, Orff's curriculum included percussion instruments, the recorder, choreography, conducting, chorus, harmony, and figured bass. All of these skills were learned and practiced through improvisation. Keetman published the first recorder pieces and dance pieces based on the philosophical concepts of the school in 1930. These basic skills and concepts were demonstrated in her *Exercises in Elemental Music*, also published in 1930 (Warner, 1991).

With the help of these publications, Orff's concept of music education began to draw public attention, and by 1931, it had gained popularity. Plans to incorporate Orff Schulwerk into public schools were made but halted by the political turmoil of 1930s Germany. In 1933, Orff could no longer fund his work. Many of his publications were forced out of print due to political controversy. Over the next several years, Orff withdrew from working at the school. The school was closed for political reasons in 1944 and destroyed a year later by bombings. During these difficult years, Orff was asked to compose music for the opening ceremony of the 1936 Olympic Games in Berlin. Although somewhat antithetical to his philosophy, he created processional music and a group dance for thousands of young children. This drew the attention of a German administrator who, in 1948, questioned whether his music could be played by the children themselves. This sparked interest and led Orff to change his focus to incorporate more singing and children's songs and to design instruments appropriately sized for children. Thus began the second phase of the Schulwerk.

This second phase of Schulwerk led to the refinement of Orff's education program. With Keetman's help, Orff renewed his attempt to reform music education after being asked to participate in radio broadcasts of children's programs. The Bavarian Broadcasting Company approached him to create these programs, with the first broadcast airing September 1948. Because much of the material from the Guntherschule had been destroyed, Orff enlisted Klauss Becker, a pupil of Karl Maendler, to put together the xylophones and metallophones of the new Schulwerk (Orff, 1963).

In 1949, Keetman began teaching courses for children at the Academie der Tonkunst Mozarteum in Salzburg, Austria. The courses were based on the radio broadcasts but now included the element of movement deemed essential to the Schulwerk. These courses continued to be a huge success in the field of music education.

It was not until the early 1950s that the concepts of Orff Schulwerk were written down. Beginning in 1950, Orff and Keetman spent 4 years writing down the concepts they had developed throughout their experiences. They published *Music for Children* in five volumes and promoted the concept of a music education program based on "music meant for and created by children." Orff training programs started in 1953 at the Mozarteum in Salzburg. Ten years later, the program outgrew the Mozarteum, and the Orff Institute was founded just outside of Salzburg (Warner, 1991).

Orff Schulwerk continued to gain popularity around the world, making it one of the most well-known approaches of music education. Its spread to other countries began in 1953 with a presentation at the International Conference of Directors of Music Academies, which was held at the Mozarteum. Several of Orff's students introduced the idea of elemental music to music directors and educators through demonstration of the Orff Schulwerk curriculum. In 1962, Orff, Keetman, and several of their students taught the first course of Orff training in North America in Toronto, Ontario, Canada. Over the next several years, Orff Schulwerk spread across North America, and in 1968, the American Orff-Schulwerk Association was founded. *Music for Children* was eventually translated into English, and by 1956 and 1982, the first three volumes had been published in Canada and the United States, respectively (Shamrock, 1997). The understanding is that each culture should use its own speech and song heritage as the basis for the approach. Methods of Orff Schulwerk are now incorporated into music education programs across North America (Frazee & Kreuter, 1987; Warner, 1991).

Orff Schulwerk and Music Therapy

Carl Orff did not design the Orff Schulwerk approach for music therapy, and no documented records show him adapting his curriculum to children with any specific disabilities. He does make reference to music therapy in a translated speech made at the opening session of the Orff elementary education course at the University of Toronto in 1962. He states that "the growing interest in the Schulwerk, the editing just mentioned, the additions of whole new fields such as music therapy, kept me extremely busy" (Orff, 1963, p. 74). Later, in a 1964 speech, Orff stated:

> The child and the common man are still creatures who are attuned to the powers of rhythm. They prove in their joy . . . in their dance as well as their work, that rhythm is a gift that makes her dearest children happy, and gives strength to the most tormented of them. (Orff, 1994, p. 13)

Beginning in 1962, Wilhelm Keller, who was serving as director of the Orff Institute in Salzburg, applied the techniques of the Orff Schulwerk to exceptional populations. He worked with children with emotional disturbances in Austria, with students with mental and physical disabilities in a special school in Salzburg, and later with young adults diagnosed with Down syndrome, spastic paralysis, mental retardation, and/or severe disabilities (Lehrer-Carle, 1971).

Despite potentially no direct attention given by Orff himself, many of the principles of Orff Schulwerk can be applied to various populations of clients in music therapy. One of the first documented adaptations of the Orff approach was in 1969 by Judith Bevans. She worked at a school for children who were blind, and her program was based on the fundamental assumption that "all children possess, in different degrees, the abilities to be creative and to express themselves" (Bevans, 1969, p. 41). Since then, Orff Schulwerk has been integrated into music therapy and education programs for many different clients (Adelman, 1979; Ball & Bitcon, 1974; Barker, 1981; Bernstorf, 1997; Birkenshaw-Fleming, 1997; Burns, 1987; Dervan, 1982; Ellin, 1991 Hochheimer, 1976; Hollander & Juhrs, 1974; Leonard, 1997; Levine, 1998; McRae, 1982; Nordlund, 1997; Orff, 1994; Ponath & Bitcon, 1972). The most notable publications devoted solely to the topic of Orff Music Therapy are by Gertrud Orff—*The Orff Music Therapy: Active Furthering of the Development of the Child* (1974) and *Key Concepts in the Orff Music Therapy* (1989), and by Carol Bitcon—*Alike and Different: The Clinical and Educational Uses of Orff Schulwerk* (2000).

Philosophy

General Philosophy of Orff Schulwerk

At the core of Orff Schulwerk lie two basic premises: that everyone is able to participate in music, and that the music used in the classroom must be elemental in nature. Regardless of ability or disability, every child in the Orff ensemble participates. This may take the form of speech, singing, instrument playing, or movement. The teacher must serve as a guide, placing children in parts they are able to successfully perform (Colwell, 2005; Shamrock, 1997; Warner, 1991).

At the heart of Orff instruction is elemental music. As stated, this music is "primal" in nature and integrates the elements of speech, dance, and movement. Orff believed that this music must never stand alone, as this is not how it is treated in tribal cultures (Orff, 1994). This music is not meant to be written and strictly performed. Instead, it is a process, with the musical product always allowing for change through improvisation (Rudaitis, 1995; Warner, 1991).

One of the guiding principles behind the Orff approach to music education is the progression from sound to symbol. Orff believed that this progression of music learning paralleled that of language acquisition in children. Therefore, the approach was developed to support this premise. As children learn language, we surround them with the tools to learn the language: spoken conversation, affirmation of their attempts, and pictorial and textual contexts. In the Schulwerk approach, children participate in a myriad of music making before they verbalize the experience (Wry, 1981). Children learn the sounds of music and words initially (exploration and imitation), and then begin to manipulate them through harmony and sentence formation (improvisation and creation). Children are only gradually introduced to the written form (of music or text) once they have a firm grasp on the sounds used. As children become more comfortable with reading, they are eventually asked to create through music or textual writing (Bitcon, 2000; Orff, 1963).

Through this progression from sound to symbol, the Schulwerk provides for the development of musical concepts. Rhythm is considered the foundation for all further work and is the strength and unifying force in elemental music (speech, dance, and movement). From speech, children move into the development of melody (call and response, chanting, pentatonic modes, and diatonic modes) as well as further development of unmetered and metered speech. Movement expands into three areas of conceptual development: rhythmic movement, free/interpretive movement, and accompaniment. Accompaniment becomes an integral component of the process of Orff Schulwerk. Children begin to use unpitched instruments, followed by pitched instruments to accompanying their speech, singing, and movement activities. This development of accompaniment skills eventually leads to an understanding of traditional harmony. Throughout this process, movement continues to be used to model accompaniment patterns from the simple bordun to a rhythmic ostinato used as color (Morin, 1996; Warner, 1991).

In 1980, Coralie Snell completed her dissertation, *The Philosophical Basis of Orff Schulwerk*. Through an analysis of the literature and other pertinent sources, she summarized the belief system of Schulwerk proponents to nine basic points:

1. Education should provide opportunities for experiences that lead to the full development of each individual according to his/her specific needs, abilities, and potentialities.
2. The power to create is an inherent characteristic of all human beings.
3. The potential for expressiveness lies within each person and will respond to the right stimulation.
4. Pleasurable experience enhances any learning and tends to provide greater retention of that learning.
5. Learning in general, and music learning in particular, should come about as the result of participation in experiences, which lead toward that learning.
6. Music is essential to the total development of human beings.
7. The learning of music theory is a direct outgrowth of continuous participation in Orff Schulwerk experiences.
8. The best way for children to learn music is through the repetition of the historical process by which humanity has acquired its own present musicality.
9. The group is important and each individual has a unique contribution to make to the group.

Orff-Based Music Therapy

Much of Orff's philosophy of music education parallels that of music therapy. Several aspects of the Orff Schulwerk approach support music therapy. These include allowing everyone to participate in music, beginning where the individual is developmentally, using a multisensory approach, using rhythm as the underlying foundation of elemental music, moving from the experiential to the conceptual, designing experiences that are success-oriented, using culturally specific material, and focusing on the process rather than the product (Colwell, 2005).

Orff felt that everyone should be allowed to participate in the musical experience (Shamrock, 1997). Therapeutic change occurs when the client is engaged in the session and the opportunity for participation in Orff orchestrations at a myriad of levels provides the opportunity for all clients to participate.

Orff felt that the approach should begin where the child is developmentally and musically (Orff, 1963). Crucial to Orff-based Music Therapy is a tenet well known to music therapists: start where the client is and focus on what he or she can do (iso principle). The therapist must be flexible and adapt music therapy applications to tap into these abilities of clients while also working toward established goals. Accompanying musical learning and development must be tailored to the client's pace and be very individualized. In Orff, this is described as an alternation between tension and release. This involves careful combinations of novelty and familiarity while avoiding routine. Changes made build interest both within the session and between sessions, which may be termed "fascination" in Orff Music Therapy (Orff, 1974).

One of the most important of these common aspects is the multisensory approach. Orff's goal of reaching every child is manifested through the use of several sense modalities to increase the likelihood of learning. Speech, singing, movement, and playing instruments, the core components of the Orff Schulwerk, shape this multisensory approach. For example, instruments may reach clients on a tactile, visual, auditory, or kinesthetic level. Clients may respond to the texture or weight of an instrument, to its size and color, to its timbre, or to the movement required to elicit a sound (Orff, 1974). Orff believed rhythm is the foundation of elemental music providing the underpinning for these multisensory experiences. Analogous to this view, Gaston (1968) believed that rhythm is the energizer and organizer in music and thus was the impetus for the therapeutic change through music.

As discussed previously, one of Orff's guiding principles is the progression from sound to symbol or from the experiential to the conceptual (Wry, 1981). Therapeutic intervention in music therapy grows out of attention to the functional outcome. The musical experience is designed based on this goal with the understanding that the client may not always be aware of the intent of the experience during music participation. Orff felt strongly that these musical experiences should be designed such that they are success-oriented (Bitcon, 2000) and use culturally specific material (Warner, 1991). In therapy, if clients are positive about an experience using culturally familiar and preferred music, there is likely to be increased engagement, desire for repetition, motivation to change, and potential progress toward the therapeutic goal.

While the primary goal of music education and music therapy differ (music vs. nonmusic outcomes), the focus on the process of the musical experience rather than on the end musical product is comparable (Shamrock, 1997). In therapy, the intended goal is a functional outcome for the client in a variety of domain areas (i.e., motor, communication, cognitive) with therapeutic change occurring as a result of the process of a musical application or intervention. Orff felt that musical learning occurred as a result of the process of participation in the musical experience rather than as a result of the end musical product (Colwell, 2005).

In her book, *Alike and Different: The Clinical and Educational Uses of Orff Schulwerk*, Carol Bitcon (2000) lists four underlying premises when working with the Orff Schulwerk in clinical settings. First, success must be implicit in the session. The environment should be positive and nonthreatening and create a mood for risk taking. Clients should be willing to take chances with successive approximations rewarded. Second, open-ended material should be presented to whatever degree possible. Although the therapist may have a specific goal in mind, he or she must allow for variation on that response by the client. Depending upon the ability level of the client, the amount of control the therapist initiates will vary. Third, materials used must be appropriate to the abilities of the individuals in the group. Somewhat self-explanatory, the therapist should use material developmentally appropriate to the clients to ensure success (the first premise). Last, adaptability, flexibility, sensitivity, knowledge of disabilities and therapeutic needs, a sense of humor, and a regard for personal dignity must be employed.

Clinical Applications of Music Therapy

The Orff Schulwerk pedagogy focuses on leading children through four areas of musical development: exploration, imitation, improvisation and creation. The first area is exploration, whereby children discover the realm of possibilities in sound and movement. Children are presented a musical stimulus and given the freedom to manipulate the music. The next area is imitation. Imitation develops basic skills in the following areas: speech, body percussion, movement, singing, and playing instruments. The teacher or therapist presents a pattern and asks children to repeat it. This may be done informally or in a call and response form. Regardless of presentation, the area of imitation should first be presented through body percussion (snapping, clapping, stomping, or patschen), and then be transferred to either nonpitched percussion, pitched percussion (xylophones, glockenspiels, metallophones), or the recorder. The areas of exploration and imitation are often introduced simultaneously or interchangeably dependent upon the context.

Once children are able to imitate patterns correctly, the therapist introduces improvisation. Improvisation focuses on the skill areas targeted for imitation such as body percussion, while providing opportunities for the individual to initiate new patterns. The child can participate in the group activity using whatever level of improvisation skills he or she has attained. Improvisation is introduced as soon as children are able to imitate even the most basic patterns. The teacher or therapist structures improvisation, encouraging children to alter either the rhythm or pitches of previously learned material. This may take the form of question and answer, or a rondo form in which solo playing alternates with group playing.

The final area is creation. In this stage, the group combines material from the first three areas of exploration, imitation, and improvisation. Children are encouraged to create their own works in the form of rondos, theme and variations, or mini-suites. The text may be original or borrowed from material holding special meaning for the "composer" and may be musically developed through using the core components of the Orff Schulwerk approach: speech, singing, movement, and/or playing instruments (Shamrock, 1997).

Throughout this process, the Orff Schulwerk approach teaches musical and aesthetic responsiveness. Children learn to think deeply and to respond and express themselves in ways unique to the arts. Musical responsiveness includes sensory awareness, aesthetic experience, skill development, and improvisation. Orff activities stimulate the child's various senses, that is, auditory, tactile, visual, and kinesthetic). Children have opportunities to be expressive, creative, and imaginative while participating with their whole bodies. During Orff Schulwerk, children gain an understanding of music and nonmusic concepts through active engagement in the process through speech, singing, movement, and playing instruments (Banks, 1982; Thomas, 1980). As conceptual understanding develops, children participate in improvisation experiences through "designing, redesigning, reconstructing, rearranging, symbolizing and extending the elements" (Thomas, 1980, p. 58).

Orff felt that this approach to music making should be appropriate for music education internationally. A basic premise of the Orff Schulwerk is that the music used in these various stages of musical development begin with each culture's own speech and song heritage, including rhymes, proverbs, children's chants, games, and songs. The Orff Schulwerk approach is process-oriented; it is not product-driven (Shamrock, 1997). What happens during the music making is more important than the resulting musical product, which makes this approach ideal for the nonmusical goal-directed area of music therapy.

In her 1979 master's thesis, Adelman examined *An Integration of Music Therapy Theory and Orff Schulwerk Techniques in Clinical Application.* She applied the Orff Schulwerk approach to the "Processes in Music Therapy" outlined by William Sears (1968). These processes in music therapy are divided into three main headings: (a) Experience within structure, (b) Experience in self-organization, and (c) Experience in relating to others. Music has structure. It occurs in relation to time, is not static, and changes from moment to moment. The Orff Schulwerk is an evolving process that provides structure (such as the common rondo form) while allowing for change within the ongoing composition process (improvisation and creation). The music therapist strives to provide clients opportunities for self-motivation and personal choice as a means to self-organization and self-expression. Essential to the Orff Schulwerk process is the client's participation in the development of the composition through improvisation. Choices based on instrumentation, form, patterns, tempo, dynamics, and so forth, are critical elements of creation. Experience relating to others is integral to successful music making. Because the Orff Schulwerk composition relies on the pulse ostinato and often an underlying rhythmic ostinato, the individual members of the group must strive for group cohesion as well as strength of independence as they fit their individual parts into the orchestration (Adelman, 1979).

The clinical use of Orff Schulwerk in music education and therapy settings has been primarily used with children but has expanded to other populations in recent years. Articles have been written that focus on the use of the Orff Schulwerk with specific populations in music education mainstreamed or inclusion settings (Crinklaw-Kiser, 1996; Hunter, 1997; Velasquez, 1997) as well as in therapeutic settings (Burnett, 1994; Cole, 1998; Ellin, 1991; Gadberry, 2005). Those populations include autism (Benedict, 1984); hearing impaired (Birkenshaw-Fleming, 1997; Campbell, 1979); gifted (Gregoire, Hughes, Robbins, & Voorneveld, 1989); learning disabled (Baird, 1982; Barker, 1981; Beck, 1985); developmentally disabled (Baxter, 1972); neurological disorders (Bernstorf, 1997); and orthopedically impaired (Nordlund, 1997). While the contextual setting may have been the music education classroom, these articles reflect the understanding that, when working with children with special needs, the focus expands beyond music skills to nonmusical outcomes.

Outside of the elementary music classroom, the Orff Schulwerk approach has been modified to be used with children with behavior disorders (Whittington, 2008); psychiatric patients (Levine, 1998); child bereavement groups (Hilliard, 2007); well-elderly (Gray, 1981; Ernst, 2003; Margeson, 1973; Peters, 2004; Richardson, 2000, 2003, 2008); and intergenerational groups (Sabourin, 2000; Shotwell, 1985).

Within Orff-based Music Therapy, music is seen as having many functions to address change in a variety of targeted domain areas. Examples could be in social and communication domains.

Participation in an Orff ensemble gives the client a sense of identity as a participant whose presence is needed in the ensemble. The therapy acts as a stimulus, creating a sense of belonging and of contribution to something larger: the total music product (Orff, 1974). The need for cooperation and turn taking in these ensembles builds the capacity to tolerate others. Consequently, playing in these ensembles may increase a client's ability to react to and interact with others.

The Orff instrumentarium also allows for several forms of communication. Instruments may dually serve as a link and as a barrier between client and therapist. The client can communicate intentions to the therapist through playing the instrument but may also use it to create a "safe" distance between therapist and client (Orff, 1974). Thus, communication may take place from the child to the instrument, from the child to the therapist, and (in group settings) from client to client.

When completing a music therapy assessment as a precursor to designing a treatment plan for any of these client populations, the following areas may be considered as potential targets: social, communication, motor, cognitive, psychological, perception of self, reality awareness, emotional, vision, hearing, and music. Table 1 provides just a few of the many applications of the Orff Schulwerk process when working on the essential nonmusical and music goals commonly found in a music therapy treatment plan. The table lists the target area, specific behaviors associated with that area, and the possibilities for Orff applications.

Summary

Although Carl Orff did not purposely establish his approach as a protocol for music therapy, the approach he developed is easily incorporated into music therapy sessions. Since many of the goals are the same, the underlying principles are also similar. At the basis of Orff Schulwerk is the ability for music to speak through its expression, and it is through this expression that music can address the therapeutic goals. According to Bevans (1969), Orff Schulwerk embodies the fundamental principles that "rhythm is present in all of life" and that "very few children are a-musical" (p. 42). By adopting these principles, the approach of Orff can be applied to any population served by music therapists.

Table 1

Orff Applications for Targeted Behaviors

Targeted Areas	Specific Behaviors	Orff Applications
Social	Taking turns Following directions	Imitation, Solo/Ensemble playing Ostinatos, Rhythmic dancing
Communication	Using speech Question–Answer skills	Chants, Speech ostinatos Call and response activities
Motor	Motor imitation Palmar grasp	Body percussion imitation/ostinatos Mallet positioning and use
Cognitive	Listening skills Recognizes name	Rote teaching of ensemble parts Myriad of name games and chants
Psychological	Stress release Self-control	Improvisation, Free movement Creation choices, Participation level
Perception of self	Verbal expression of self Body language presentation	Create chants describing self Mirroring movement to increase comfort
Reality awareness	Name recognition Sequencing of daily events	Theme and variations: Child and information Barred accompaniment to original song
Emotional	Expression of feelings Distinguishing emotions	Improvisation, Composition, Singing Create work based on an emotion
Vision	Visual tracking Symbol/Letter discrimination	Reading charts for rhythms/text Rondo activities using visuals
Hearing	Auditory discrimination Peer interaction	Environmental sounds in composition Ensemble performance
Music	Anything	And everything!

References

Adelman, E. J. (1979). An integration of music therapy theory and Orff Schulwerk techniques in clinical application (Master's thesis, Michigan State University, 1979). *Masters Abstracts International, 18*(2).

American Orff-Schulwerk Association (AOSA). (2000, October 8). *Chronology of Orff Schulwerk.* Retrieved from http://www.aosa.org/chronology.html

Baird, D. P. (1982). The learning disabled child in the Orff classroom: Jumping head first into the mainstream. *The Orff Echo, 4*(3), 5, 9–11.

Ball, T. S., & Bitcon, C. H. (1974). Generalized imitation and Orff Schulwerk. *Mental Retardation, 12*(3), 36–39.

Banks, S. (1982). Orff Schulwerk teaches musical responsiveness. *Music Educators Journal, 68*(7), 42–43.

Barker, C. S. (1981). Using Orff Schulwerk as a method to enhance self concept in children with learning disabilities (Doctoral dissertation, Brigham Young University, 1981). *Dissertation Abstracts International, 42*(05A).

Baxter, C. M. (1972). Orff with the retarded. *The Orff Echo, 4*(2), 3–4.

Beck, M. (1985). Music, movement, and the learning disabled child. *The Orff Echo, 17*(4), 5–8.

Benedict, R. E. (1984). The autistic child. *The Orff Echo, 16*(4), 13, 20.

Bernstorf, E. (1997). Orff Schulwerk, inclusion and neurological disorders. *The Orff Echo, 29*(2), 8–11.

Bevans, J. (1969). The exceptional child and Orff. *Music Educators Journal, 55*(7), 41–43, 125–127.

Birkenshaw-Fleming, L. (1997). The Orff approach and the hearing impaired. *The Orff Echo, 29*(2), 15–19.

Bitcon, C. H. (2000). *Alike and different: The clinical and educational uses of Orff Schulwerk* (2nd ed.). Gilsum, NH: Barcelona.

Burnett, M. (1994). The roots of Orff Schulwerk in music therapy. *The Orff Echo, 26*(4), 10.

Burns, K. (1987). Orff Schulwerk in an instititutional setting. *The Orff Echo, 19*(3), 24–25.

Campbell, C. (1979). Coming together through music: Integration of hearing and hearing-impaired children. *The Orff Echo, 11*(4), 9–10.

Carl Orff Foundation. (1999, February 22). *Carl Orff 1895–1982*. Retrieved from http://orff.munich. netsurf.de/orff/html_e/body_leben_und_werk.html

Cole, J. (1998). Playing mallet instruments: Some motor skill development considerations. *The Orff Echo,* 10–12.

Colwell, C. M. (2005). An Orff approach to music therapy. *The Orff Echo, 38*(1), 19–21.

Crinklaw-Kiser, D. (1996). Integrating music with whole language through the Orff Schulwerk process. *Young Children, 51*(5), 15–21.

Dervan, N. (1982). Building Orff ensemble skills with mentally handicapped adolescents. *Music Educators Journal, 68*(8), 35–36, 60–61.

Ellin, B. (1991). Music with the visually impaired. *The Orff Echo, 24*(1), 20–21.

Ernst, R. (2003). Orff Schulwerk for senior adults. *The Orff Echo, 35*(2), 28–31.

Frazee, J., & Kreuter, K. (1987). *Discovering Orff*. New York: Schott Music.

Gadberry, A. (2005). Reaching students with special needs through the Orff approach. *The Orff Echo, 38*(1), 27–31.

Gaston, E. T. (1968). *Music in therapy*. New York: Macmillan.

Gray, E. C. (1981). Fokan: Musical exercises for health and well-being for older adulthood. *The Orff Echo, 14*(1), 5–7.

Gregoire, M. A., Hughes, J. E., Robbins, B. J., & Voorneveld, R. B. (1989). Music therapy with the gifted? A trial program. *Music Therapy Perspective, 7*, 23–27.

Hilliard, R.E. (2007). The effects of Orff-based music therapy and social work groups on childhood grief symptoms and behaviors. *Journal of Music Therapy, 44*, 123–138.

Hochheimer, L. (1976). Musically planned creativity and flexibility—elementary classroom: Implications for Orff Schulwerk, the Kodály methods and music therapy. *Creative Child and Adult Quarterly, 1*(4), 200–206.

Hollander, F. M., & Juhrs, P. D. (1974). Orff Schulwerk: An effective treatment tool with autistic children. *Journal of Music Therapy, 11,* 1–12.

Hunter, B. C. (1997). Inclusion in the music classroom or inclusive music instruction? *The Orff Echo, 29*(2), 28–29, 31.

Lehrer-Carle, I. (1971). Orff Schulwerk: A vitalizing tool in music therapy programs. *Musart, 23,* 10.

Leonard, S. F. (1997). Special songs, special kids: Learning opportunities for the special learner. *The Orff Echo, 29*(2), 20–21.

Levine, C. (1998). Reminiscences: Orff Schulwerk at the Detroit Psychiatric Institute. *The Orff Echo, 30,* 30–32.

Margeson, F. (1973). Our senior citizens. *The Orff Echo, 5*(2), 1, 3, 6.

McRae, S. W. (1982). The Orff connection. Reaching the special child. *Music Educators Journal, 68*(8), 32–34.

Morin, F. (1996). *The Orff Schulwerk movement: A case study in music education reform.* (ERIC Document Reproduction Service No. ED 420 608)

Nordlund, S. (1997). Me? Work with orthopedically what? *The Orff Echo, 29*(2), 12–13.

Orff, C. (1963). Schulwerk: Its origin and aims. *Music Educators Journal, 49*(5), 69–74.

Orff, C. (1994). The Schulwerk and music therapy: Carl Orff, 1964. *The Orff Echo, 26*(4), 10–13.

Orff, G. (1974). *The Orff music therapy: Active furthering of the development of the child.* London: Schott.

Orff, G. (1989). *Key concepts in the Orff music therapy* (J. Day & S. Salmon, Trans.). London: Schott.

Peters, K. (2004). *An examination of the adult learners emotional and intellectual responses to an Orff Schulwerk music learning experience.* Unpublished master's thesis, University of St. Thomas.

Ponath, L. H., & Bitcon, C. H. (1972). A behavioral analysis of Orff Schulwerk. *Journal of Music Therapy, 9,* 56–63.

Richardson, M. L. (2000). Learning music a new way—Orff for adults. *The Orff Echo, 33*(1), 33.

Richardson, M. L. (2003). An Orff program for adults. *The Orff Echo, 35*(2), 32–33.

Richardson, M. L. (2008). Swing ensemble for pitched percussion: A new paradigm for Orff Schulwerk with senior adults. *The Orff Echo, 40*(2), 9–13.

Rudaitis, C. (1995). Jump ahead and take the risk. *Teaching Music, 2*(5), 34–35.

Sabourin, D. (2000). Sharing in process: Orff Schulwerk in intergenerational settings. *The Orff Echo, 32*(2), 24–32.

Sears, W. (1968). Processes in music therapy. In E. Thayer Gaston (Ed.), *Music in therapy* (pp. 30–46). New York: Macmillan.

Shamrock, M. (1997). Orff Schulwerk: An integrated foundation. *Music Educators Journal, 83*(6), 41–44.

Shotwell, R. (1985). Inter-generational programs. *The Orff Echo, 18*(1), 25.

Snell, C. A. (1980). The philosophical basis of Orff Schulwerk (Doctoral dissertation, University of Southern California, 1980). *Dissertation Abstracts International, 41*(04A).

Thomas, J. (1980). Orff-based improvisation. *Music Educators Journal, 66*(5), 58–61.

Velasquez, V. (1997). Exceptional populations. *The Orff Echo, 29*, 7.

Warner, B. (1991). *Orff Schulwerk: Applications for the classroom.* Englewood Cliffs, NJ: Prentice-Hall.

Whittington, D. (2008). Finding a musical voice of cooperation and teamwork: Teaching in a children's home. *The Orff Echo, 40*(2), 34–37.

Wry, O. E. (1981). Philosophical implications of Orff Schulwerk. *The Orff Echo, 13*(4), 5, 23.

Applications for the Classroom

Frazee, J., & Kreuter, K. (1987). *Discovering Orff.* New York: Schott Music.

Goodkin, D. (2002). *Play, sing, and dance: An introduction to Orff Schulwerk.* Miami, FL: Schott Music.

Keller, W. (1974). *Orff Schulwerk: Introduction to music for children* (methodology, playing the instruments, suggested for teachers). Miami, FL: European American Music Distribution Cooperation.

Landis, B., & Carder, P. (1972). *The eclectic curriculum in American music education: Contributions of Dalcroze, Kodaly, and Orff.* Washington, DC.: Music Educators National Conference.

Nash, G. C. (1974). *Creative approaches to child development with music, language, and movement.* Port Washington, NY: Alfred.

Regner, H. (Coordinator). (1977, 1980, 1982). *Music for children. Orff Schulwerk American edition* (Vols. 1–3). New York: Schott Music.

Saliba, K. K. (1991). *Accent on Orff: An introductory approach.* Englewood Cliffs, NJ: Prentice-Hall.

Steen, A. (1992). *Exploring Orff: A teacher's guide.* New York: Schott Music.

Warner, B. (1991). *Orff Schulwerk: Applications for the classroom.* Englewood Cliffs, NJ: Prentice-Hall.

Wheeler, L., & Raebeck, L. (1985). *Orff and Kodaly adapted for the elementary school.* Dubuque, IA: Wm. C. Brown.

Additional Resources

American Orff-Schulwerk Association (AOSA). Website: http://www.aosa.org/

Carl Orff Canada. Website: http://www.orffcanada.ca/

The Orff Echo. Quarterly publication of the AOSA.

Ostinato. Publication of COC, published three times per year.

Selected Orff Schulwerk Collections

Dupont, D., & Hiller, B. (2004). *It's elemental* (1 and 2). Lakeland, TN: Memphis Musicraft.

Dupont, D., & Hiller, B. (2005). *Earth, water, fire, air! A suite for voices, narrator and Orff instruments.* Lakeland, TN: Memphis Musicraft.

Dupont, D., & Hiller, B. (2008). *Make a joyful sound! A celebration of Orff Schulwerk media.* Lakeland, TN: Memphis Musicraft.

Ferguson, N. (1987). *Good morning John Denver: Denver's greatest hits arranged for elementary singers.* Memphis, TN: Memphis Musicraft.

Forrest, L. (1994). *Orffestrations.* Dayton, OH: Heritage Music Press. (Various volumes focusing on different topics)

Frazee, J. (1983). *Singing in the season.* St Louis, MO: MMB Music.

Hampton, W. (1995). *Hot marimba.* Danbury, CT: World Music Press.

Judah-Lauder, C. (2001). *Hand drums on the move.* Bridgewater, VA: Beatin' Path.

Judah-Lauder, C. (2004). *To drum.* Bridgewater, VA: Beatin' Path.

Kriske, J., & Delelles, R. (1999). *Strike it rich!* Las Vegas, NV: Kid Sounds.

McRae, S. W. (1980). *Chatter with the angels.* St. Louis, MO: MMB Music.

McRae, S. W. (1982). *Glow ree bee.* Lakeland, TN: Memphis Musicraft.

McRae, S. W. (1985). *American sampler.* Lakeland, TN: Memphis Musicraft.

McRae, S. W. (1992). *Playtime.* Memphis, TN: Memphis Musicraft.

McRae, S. W. (1995). *Sing 'round the world.* Lakeland, TN: Memphis Musicraft.

McRae, S. W. (2003). *Homespun: Folksongs of rural America.* Lakeland, TN: Memphis Musicraft.

Memphis Orff Teachers. (1981). *Hearing America.* Memphis, TN: Memphis Musicraft.

Memphis Orff Teachers. (1991). *The world sings.* Lakeland, TN: Memphis Musicraft.

Mueller, S. (2008). *Simply speaking.* Bridgewater, VA: Beatin' Path.

Nash, G. C., & Rapley, J. (1990). *Music in the making.* Van Nuys, CA: Alfred.

Olsen, A. (1987). *13 songs for Halloween.* Vancover, WA: Alice Olsen.

Saliba, K. (1981). *Who's who at the zoo?* Cordova, TN: Cock-A-Doodle Tunes.

Saliba, K. (1982). *Jelly beans and things.* Memphis, TN: Memphis Musicraft.

Saliba, K. (1993). *Yours truly. Creative choices for Orff classrooms.* Memphis, TN: Memphis Musicraft.

Saliba, K. (1994). *One world, many voices.* Memphis, TN: Memphis Musicraft.

Saliba, K. (1995a). *Good morning songs and wake-up games.* Lakeland, TN: Memphis Musicraft.

Saliba, K. (1995b). *Sing me a song.* Miami, FL: Warner Bros.

Saliba, K. (1996). *Austinato: An ostinato jamboree.* Lakeland, TN: Memphis Musicraft.

Saliba, K. (1998a). *Spice it up.* Miami, FL: Warner Bros.

Saliba, K. (1998b). *With a twist.* Lakeland, TN: Memphis Musicraft.

Saliba, K. (1999). *Pot-pourri.* Miami, FL: Warner Bros.

Chapter 3

The Dalcroze Approach to Music Therapy

R. J. David Frego
Robin E. Liston
Mika Hama
Greta Gillmeister

Introduction

The Dalcroze approach to music education and therapy is based on contributions from the Swiss musician and educator, Émile-Henri Jaques-Dalcroze. The approach is somatic in that the activities and games are focused to connect the brain with the body and the emotional spirit of creativity and the nuances of music. It centers on an idea that has been valued at various times throughout history, that the synthesis of the mind, the body, and the emotions is fundamental to all learning. Plato said in his *Laws*: "Education has two branches, one of gymnastics, which is concerned with the body and the other of music, which is designed for the improvement of the soul" (Pennington, 1925, p. 9). Jaques-Dalcroze believed that the goal of every musician is to be sensitive and expressive, and to express music through movement, sound, thought, feeling, and creation.

Three facets of Dalcroze Eurhythmics are layered upon each other to create the approach. These are eurhythmics, which is centered in purposeful movement and is often described as the most visible component; *solfège rhythmique,* which is both physical and vocal and is designed to develop inner hearing; and improvisation, which transfers the learning from movement improvisation to instrumental and vocal improvisation.

Mead (1994) describes the Dalcroze approach in terms of four basic premises:

1. Eurhythmics awakens physical, aural, and visual images of music in the mind.
2. *Solfège* (sight-singing and ear training), improvisation, and eurhythmics together work to improve expressive musicality and enhance intellectual understanding.
3. Music may be experienced through speech, gesture, and movement. These can likewise be experienced in time, space, and energy.

4. Humans learn best when learning through the senses. Music should be taught through the tactile, the kinesthetic, the aural, and the visual senses.

History

Émile-Henri Jaques was born into a musical home on July 6, 1865. His Swiss parents were living in Vienna, and young Émile and his sister Hélène were supported in their artistic education by their mother Julie, herself a fine music teacher and pianist. She had studied the philosophy and teaching approaches of educational reformer Heinrich Pestalozzi (1746–1827). He was an early advocate of teaching through the senses and through experience, not merely through the written word. He also supported the addition of vocal music instruction to school curricula. Pestalozzi's influence on Madame Jaques was evident in her son as well. Since the Dalcroze approach centers on the philosophy that experience in music is key to musical understanding, it seems that both Pestalozzi and Dalcroze philosophies share common ground (Collins, 1993). Childhood in the Jaques household was a time of singing, playing, dancing, acting, and creating. Émile had a happy childhood and was described as "lively, friendly, and even contemplative for a child" (Spector, 1990, p. 5).

In 1875, the family returned to Geneva. After several years in a private school, Émile Jaques enrolled at the Geneva Conservatory. At the age of 18, he had not yet decided upon a career. The following year, 1884, he went to Paris, where he studied drama at the *Comédie Française* and music at the Paris Conservatory. Young Émile reveled in the artistic atmosphere of the city. A passionate young actor and musician, he also found time to compose and perform, singing as he accompanied himself on the piano.

While in Paris, Émile Jaques became familiar with the teachings of Mathis Lussy (1828–1910), a piano instructor and writer. Lussy wrote extensively on the subject of expressive musical performance and musical understanding (Caldwell, 1995). Through Lussy, Émile Jaques learned of the process of scholarly inquiry: to recognize problems, to approach them scientifically, and to devise methods for their solution (Spector, 1990). Émile Jaques' interests were shifting toward an emphasis in music, and after a visit with his family in Geneva in the summer of 1886, he accepted the position of assistant conductor and chorus master at the Théâtre des Nouveaux in Algiers, North Africa. Algeria had been a French colony since 1847 and consequently felt the influence of Western European culture. Émile Jaques underwent two changes while enjoying his first professional employment. Feeling that his youthful appearance might inhibit his effectiveness as a leader, he began sporting the mustache and goatee he would maintain for the rest of his life. This was also the time when he added Dalcroze to his birth name Jaques. It seems that a composer of polkas in Bordeaux, France, also had the name Émile Jaques. To avoid confusion, Émile-Henri borrowed the name Valcroze from a friend, changed the first letter to D, and was known thereafter as Émile Jaques-Dalcroze (Spector, 1990).

After one season, Jaques-Dalcroze returned to Geneva in 1887 and, later that year, moved to Vienna and enrolled at the Vienna Conservatory in the studio of Anton Bruckner (1824–1927). Their collaboration was brief: Bruckner insisted that "der dumme Franzose" study harmony from the beginning, which Jaques-Dalcroze refused to do. Eventually Bruckner attempted to have Jaques-Dalcroze thrown out of the conservatory but was thwarted by the faculty. Adolf Prosniz (1827–1917) invited Jaques-Dalcroze into his studio. It may have been Prosniz who helped

Jaques-Dalcroze focus his musical concentration and learn to study music with greater depth (Spector, 1990). In spite of his clashes with Bruckner, Jaques-Dalcroze considered their association valuable. Bruckner's intolerance and authoritative style were the antithesis of Jaques-Dalcroze's loving, playful nature. Perhaps this experience helped to solidify his idea that an effective teacher is one who respects and educates the whole child.

Spring of 1889 brought Jaques-Dalcroze's return to the Paris Conservatory and composition study with Gabriel Fauré. The 24-year-old musician made the most of his opportunities, moving in the same musical circles as César Franck and other artists of his stature. Jaques-Dalcroze continued to compose an assortment of songs, ensembles, and sketches based on the customs of the day.

In 1892, Jaques-Dalcroze returned to the Geneva Conservatory, this time as a professor of *solfège*. He began to question the teaching approaches of the day and wonder what improvements he could make. Careful observation of his students showed him that, while the students could be good musical technicians, they often did not hear or feel the nuances of the music they were required to play. Just keeping a steady beat was often difficult for the students. Jaques-Dalcroze began by getting the students up from their seats, keeping a steady beat by moving about the space. From there he added other fundamental qualities of singing, breathing, walking at various tempi, skipping, and conducting with large gestures (Odom, 1998). He then added quality to the movement by asking them to physically react to the improvised music that he was providing at the piano. These qualities included *legato*, *marcato*, and *staccato* movements to complement the music. Cooperative work with a partner allowed the students to experience timing, space, strength and weight, creativity, and cooperative learning. By adding rhythmic movement to music, students acknowledged the body as the first instrument of expression (Dutoit, 1971, p. 9). As instructor of *solfège*, Jaques-Dalcroze believed that the compartmentalization of music courses was detrimental to the pupils' true musical development (Carder, 1990). By combining *solfège* with rhythmic movement and improvisation into *rhythmic gymnastics*, as he first called this work, Jaques-Dalcroze began to teach in a holistic style.

From 1903 to 1910, Jaques-Dalcroze actively pursued the development of a teaching approach based on rhythmic gymnastics. However, his colleagues at the Geneva Conservatory considered him something of a radical. The disapproval that met his innovations was due partly to the conservatory faculty's unwillingness to condone his experimental techniques and to have its students become "performing monkeys" (Dutoit, 1971, p. 14). Another branch of resistance was from Genevan society itself. Jaques-Dalcroze's students dressed in short-sleeved tunics, with bare legs and feet, to allow for free movement in class. This was quite an affront to most Genevans, who lived according to the rigid morality of the early 20th century. The female students were subsequently referred to by the Genevan society as *The Lost Girls* (Minder-Jeanneret, 1995).

People outside of Geneva, however, were keen to adopt Jaques-Dalcroze's approach to music and movement education. After a eurhythmics demonstration in Berlin, Jaques-Dalcroze received an offer to develop an institution for rhythmic study at an experimental garden city being designed north of Dresden, Germany. The premise of *Hellerau* was to be a community that combined a planned industrial settlement with a school for artistic development attended by children and adults. Between the years of 1910 and 1914, Hellerau became a cultural center for music, theatre, and dance.

In partnership with Adolphe Appia, a noted theatre designer, Jaques-Dalcroze supervised the construction of a school and performance space that was noted for its architectural and theatrical innovations—instead of a proscenium, the space was now open, which brought the audience closer in to the performances. In addition, all components were completely modular, which allowed the performers to move the stage in front of the audience (Spector, 1990). During performances, students were not categorized as musicians, dancers, or actors, but functioned as all three. In the summers of 1912 and 1913, audiences flocked to Hellerau to see the student summer performance of Gluck's *Orfeo ed Euridice*. These demonstrations attracted notable artists and teachers from around the world: theatre luminaries Konstantin Stanislavsky and George Bernard Shaw; dancers Mary Wigman, Sergei Diaghilev, and Rudolf von Laban; and musicians Darius Milhaud and Ignacy Jan Paderewski (Martin et al., 1965).

With the outbreak of World War I, the Hellerau school was closed and a permanent school was founded in Geneva. Jaques-Dalcroze, recognizing the need for qualified instructors, designed a professional training curriculum that enabled others to teach this approach. Professional musicians and dancers at the Dalcroze School in Geneva continue to train and graduate new instructors. These graduates have established training schools in many cities around the globe (Dutoit, 1971). Jaques-Dalcroze continued writing, composing, and teaching in Geneva until his death in 1950. Besides his teaching philosophy, he is also remembered as a prolific composer of songs, operettas, and large-scale festival presentations.

Today, Dalcroze Eurhythmics is taught in music preparatory schools and is part of the music theory and aural skills curriculum in conservatories and universities throughout North America, Europe, Asia, and Australia. Training in the approach is available in the United States and in Europe. In addition, national and international professional organizations exist to support eurhythmics teachers and those interested in pursuing the experience.

Jaques-Dalcroze wanted to create an approach to music education in which sensory and intellectual experiences are fused into one neuromuscular experience—reinforcing the body's response to music (Caldwell, 1995). He felt that this would lead to performance at high levels, beyond expectation (Carder, 1990). He believed that music education should center on active involvement in musical experience. Technique and intellectual understanding are important, but active experience must come first. Today's music education is based on the "sound before the symbol" philosophy, a legacy of Jaques-Dalcroze and Pestalozzi before him. Jaques-Dalcroze felt that students could practice and learn musical expression through the active discovery of time, space, and energy. He believed that, as music moves, so should musicians; therefore, rhythm is elemental to this philosophy. Jaques-Dalcroze taught that through rhythmic movement, musicians could experience symmetry, form, tension and relaxation, phrasing, melody, and harmony. Experience should teach the musical elements.

Description

The Dalcroze approach, often identified as *Eurhythmics*, consists of three related components. The first component is *solfège rhythmique*, or ear training. Jaques-Dalcroze believed that students must learn sophisticated listening skills and develop "inner hearing." Musicians should be able to hear what they write and write what they hear. Music notation is meaningless unless realized in real performance or in the imagination. Rhythmic *solfège* is taught using the fixed-*do* approach, based on the French system. Students develop a sensitivity to pitches, their relation to each other, and to the tonal framework. What makes Dalcroze *solfège* unique is that it is always combined with rhythm and movement, both locomotor and nonlocomotor.

The second component of a Dalcroze music education is improvisation. Improvisation skills are developed sequentially and used in many ways. An instructor may play the piano while students improvise movement, react spontaneously to verbal instructions, or change in musical character. In the reverse, a student might improvise movement while another accompanies with a drum, at the piano, or in song. Students soon develop skills to be able to improvise musically and expressively on their own instruments. These spontaneous performance activities are designed to improve response time and communication accuracy (Mead, 1994).

The third aspect of the approach is the eurhythmics itself. Often considered the core of the Dalcroze approach, eurhythmics was actually the last part to be developed. Eurhythmics involves the action of participants reacting to music through purposeful and spontaneous movement. The music provided for the movement is most often improvised from the keyboard. Lessons are sequenced to allow for both discovery and success. Partner and small group activities are highlighted in order to reinforce peer learning and group collaboration. All elements of music can be presented in a eurhythmics class. However, these elements are presented in a spiral approach with increasing challenges to match the participants' progress in musical understanding and sophistication.

Educators new to eurhythmics may view the movement portion as the main descriptor. However, it is of equal importance with rhythmic *solfège* and improvisation. The term *eurhythmics* is derived from the Greek "eu," meaning good, and "rhythmy," meaning rhythm, proportion, and symmetry. This idea embodies Dalcroze philosophy in two ways. First, human beings can experience symmetry, balance, and rhythmic accuracy in music through symmetry, balance, and rhythmic accuracy in movement. Second, the three components of the Dalcroze approach (rhythmic *solfège*, improvisation, and eurhythmics) are interdependent and must be taught together. The three complement and reinforce each other, providing a complete and balanced musical education. Modern music educators and music therapists often identify the approach as *eurhythmics,* though all three facets are implied.

A typical introductory Dalcroze lesson involves activities or games that require total mental and kinesthetic awareness. The lesson is presented in a somatic approach that allows the participant to hear and react physically to the musical stimulus, which produces body awareness and sensations. These physical sensations are transmitted back to the brain as emotions and a more developed comprehension of the experience. It is common to begin a Dalcroze lesson with walking to improvised music and responding to changes in tempo, dynamics, and phrase in *quick reaction* games. Through these activities, the students begin to understand how physical adjustments, such as energy and flow of the body weight, need to occur in order to "physicalize" the music. Through these basic instructions, the teacher can address musical elements such as pulse, beat, subdivision, meter, rhythm, phrase, and form.

Intermediate Dalcroze lessons can address polymeters, polyrhythms, canon, tension and relaxation, breathing, conducting, counterpoint, and the interactions of anacrusis, crusis, and metacrusis. Creativity is pervasive throughout the lesson. All classes are in a group setting where the participants interact with partners or small groups to develop the nonverbal communication skills and creativity necessary in music and movement

Plastique Animée, or more often referred to as *plastique,* is the culminating experience in a Dalcroze class. A *plastique* combines the skills addressed throughout the class, and from previous rhythmic experiences, into a loosely based choreography that is both physically expressive and musical. The students are provided with the basics of the requirements and are asked to spontaneously create an interactive composition with the music. Someone who is stepping into a Dalcroze studio at that moment would see music in motion and might not be aware that the movement is spontaneous.

Modern music education benefits from Jaques-Dalcroze's teaching in many ways. Today's teachers focus on active learning on the part of the students. This implies less instruction and more experience for the students (Caldwell, 1993). Dalcroze philosophy also places emphasis on musical behavior and expression, and their demonstration through observable movement. Visible evidence of musical understanding through experience takes some of the mystery out of the verbal definitions of musicality and allows for informal assessment of understanding through observing movement reactions to a music stimulus.

Another aspect of modern music education inherited from Jaques-Dalcroze is the celebration of the individual. Teachers expect to provide appropriate musical experiences for all their students. Creativity and imaginary play are encouraged through improvisation. Music class is student-oriented, with groups of students actively thinking about, listening to, and analyzing and creating music (Johnson, 1993).

Dalcroze games and pedagogical principles are easy to apply to most teaching situations (Johnson, 1993). Multiage classrooms are becoming popular; Dalcroze-based activities can be adapted to suit a variety of student skill and experience levels. Dalcroze teacher training allows instructors to become creative and flexible in the give-and-take of modern education. The ability to be spontaneous in the classroom is valuable for all educators. Teachers can follow through unexpected teaching opportunities with ease and provide students with a model of an adaptable and creative personality.

Dalcroze Philosophy

Jaques-Dalcroze intended for his approach to develop musical understanding through eurhythmics and to help students develop immediate physical responsiveness to rhythmic stimuli. Developing muscular rhythms and nervous sensibility would ultimately lead to the capacity to discriminate even slight gradations of duration, time, intensity, and phrasing.

Dalcroze philosophy is centered on the interaction of time, space, and energy. The altering of one element, time, for example, creates a need to change space, and the energy to move through that space. Music is abstract; we hear it moving through time. Movement is concrete; we see it moving through space. By integrating movement with music, we begin to understand the interrelatedness of time, space, and energy. Through rhythmic movement, students would begin to think and express themselves more musically. Initially, Jaques-Dalcroze's conception of eurhythmics was designed for the education of conservatory musicians but soon expanded to the early musical education of children and to those with special needs. His philosophy grew to include his belief in the development of a more musical society through rhythmic training in the schools (Campbell, 1991).

Jaques-Dalcroze believed the learning process involved direct sensory experience. He advocated kinesthetic learning. Through movement, learning comes through experience in addition to observation. Varied musical experiences—including movement, singing, improvisation, music reading and writing, and playing instruments—reinforce musical learning (Johnson, 1993). Abramson (2001) refers to a hierarchy of learning through the Dalcroze approach: hearing to moving, moving to feeling, feeling to sensing, sensing to analyzing, analyzing to reading, reading to writing, writing to improvising, and improvising to performance. Moreover, Jaques-Dalcroze believed that the way to health was through a balance of mind, body, and senses. Many people have discovered that they can improve and refine skills by rehearsing a combination of movements, first in the real body and then imagining going through these movements with special fluidity in the kinesthetic body. One can then return to the same movement in the real body, allowing the improved flow of kinesthetic rehearsal to carry over into actual movement (Abramson, 1980).

Jaques-Dalcroze placed special emphasis on child-centered learning. He developed a particular interest in the natural development of the child (Johnson, 1993). Across ages, Jaques-Dalcroze developed music teaching strategies that were age and ability-level appropriate. His approach to music learning was broken down into experiences for the primary grades, intermediate grades, and upper grades (Mead, 1994).

Music Therapy Applications

Jaques-Dalcroze also employed the adaptation of the curriculum to the individual (Johnson, 1993). Many of the basic skills and principles of the Dalcroze approach to music education can be adapted for use in music therapy. Gaston (1968), a pioneer of music therapy, said that rhythm in music functions as the "organizer and energizer" (p. 17). This concept closely relates to Jaques-Dalcroze's eurhythmics. Music therapists can incorporate the eurhythmics portion of the Dalcroze approach by encouraging clients to move and express themselves in the process of accomplishing therapeutic goals. In addition, clinicians may study Dalcroze ideas on how to teach rhythmic concepts and adapt it for teaching children with disabilities. Jaques-Dalcroze himself adapted the approach for children with visual impairments. As mentioned previously, Jaques-Dalcroze designed several games to complement the music. Studying Dalcroze recommendations may allow clinicians to use musical games in therapeutic settings with children or adults with motor difficulties.

The hierarchy of learning, cited in the previous section, highlights the progress of hearing to moving, moving to feeling, feeling to sensing, and sensing to analyzing. This portion of the hierarchy speaks directly to goals advocated by therapists in order for clients to develop a wholeness in mind, body, and spirit.

Moreover, Jaques-Dalcroze advocated using music as a means for educating the whole child, a concept that is closely related to music therapy philosophies. The improvisational aspect of the Dalcroze approach may be useful for music therapists using Nordoff-Robbins improvisational techniques. The emphasis on rhythmic elements of music closely relates to the principles of Neurologic Music Therapy, which is discussed in another chapter in this book.

There are several accounts of music therapists incorporating Dalcroze approaches in the clinical settings. Music therapists have used eurhythmics with individuals who are HIV-positive or have AIDS-related illnesses to address their physical, mental, emotional, and social needs, and to assist in relaxation. Frego (1995) described music and movement therapy as giving palliative care to clients, in addition to helping clients take responsibility in their therapy. Music is universally available and useful, regardless of a client's disability. The goals of eurhythmics in therapy are: (a) to improve body awareness and enable clients to develop spatial awareness; (b) to bring clients to a more receptive and alert mental condition; (c) to foster creativity and imagination; (d) to integrate clients with AIDS into a group, providing verbal and physical contact with others; and (e) to provide clients with relaxation exercises and restore some personal control over their lives. Frego (1995) used an ethnographic approach in this descriptive study, relying on participant observation, informal and semistructured interviews, and literature reviews. Each session began with a relaxation exercise, followed by movement exercises accompanied by music that focused on single musical element. Clients then created a *plastique animée* (a loosely choreographed presentation). Each session ended with music-assisted relaxation. Results suggest that "music-movement therapy can provide a safe and supportive group environment that assists people to develop the social support necessary to face their future and to be able to cope creatively with their pain and apprehension" (p. 24). In addition, clients seem to develop valuable skills in maintaining some personal independence and the processing of their emotions.

More recently, Frego (2007) applied Dalcroze Eurhythmics techniques in Bosnia and Herzegovina with 12 music teachers diagnosed with post-traumatic stress disorder resulting from the civil conflict in their country. Identified characteristics prior to treatment included withdrawn behavior, social awkwardness, poor eye contact, bound movements, and extreme reactions to loud sounds. During 40 hours of Dalcroze Eurhythmics, the teacher-participants were encouraged to react to the music and use nonverbal communication and gestures in movement to communicate with partners and in small groups. Small group discussions followed each session. Throughout the process, participants showed more fluidity with their movements and a progressive connectivity with the music. Facial expression also became more evident, with increased eye contact and smiling. Common words expressed among the participants during the discussion included *release, joy, grief, loneliness*, and *tiredness*. Participants found a particular joy in connecting with other music teachers through music. As one participant stated, "It's the element that binds us all together." While this was a preliminary study, results from the discussions encourage more application of eurhythmics-type activities in group settings for those affected with PTSD.

A master's thesis investigated whether mood, focus, gross motor skills, and social interaction can be stimulated in people diagnosed with chronic schizophrenia through the use of a 6-week purposeful rhythmic movement program (Gauger, 1995). Ten patients participated in the progressive exercises that included breathing and relaxation, body awareness, rhythmic movement, group interaction, and creative movement. Data were collected through self-evaluations of mood, a rhythmic test, observation of attention and concentration, an evaluation of ward behaviors by the nurses, and video tapes. A comparison of pre- and post-evaluations reveal significant improvement in each of these areas, suggesting the need to include rhythmic movement to music in the therapy for patients with chronic schizophrenia.

Hibben (1984, 1991) reported on a program of Dalcroze eurhythmics and its effect on children with learning disabilities, emotional disturbances, or mental retardation. The researchers set several goals for the program: to mobilize the children's attention and listening skills, to help them increase their awareness of body relationships and to learn to control their movement in space, to foster peer acceptance and appreciation, and to offer opportunities for self-expression. Through music and movement games, the children explore new ideas and ultimately feel good about themselves.

A eurhythmics program for children with hearing impairments (Swaiko, 1974) emphasized such fundamentals as breath and body control, auditory training, speech improvement, creative expression, and mental health. The program focused on the creative and spontaneous expression of the child. The children worked to achieve these goals through bodily movement in speech, dance, or rhythmic improvisation. Children improved their speech production through eurhythmics, using both structured and informal approaches (Brick, 1973). Children in the primary grades participated in activities such as informal rhythm bands, creative interpretation of animals, and simple song composition. Preteen children used contrasting human voices and instrument identification to develop understanding of pitch, intensity, quality, and melodic direction in sound. Brick recommended group activities for adolescents.

Examples of Music Therapy Applications

Karen is a 6-year-old girl who exhibits behavior in the autism spectrum through a regular forward rocking motion, stimming, an aversion to loud sounds, and a negative reaction to others in close proximity. Michael, a board-certified music therapist with training in Dalcroze Eurhythmics, designs an interaction intervention to bring Karen into agreement with her behaviors and with her relation to those around her. Michael begins by softly improvising at the keyboard, using Karen's rocking motion as the tempo. By altering the tempo either slightly faster or slower, Michael is able to measure a response to Karen's awareness of the stimulus. When Karen is able to react to the tempo fluctuations, Michael starts and stops the improvisations, demonstrating different tempos and dynamics. When Michael stops playing, Karen stops rocking. In a future interaction, Michael gives Karen one end of an elastic stocking and holds the other end. A recording of improvised music programmed at Karen's preferred internal tempo is played to provide a stimulus for rhythmic swaying, dancing, and an interaction between Karen and Michael. Through additional work in rhythmic movement, Karen begins to allow rhythmic stimuli other than her own bring her closer to interactions with others.

Nell is a 48-year-old breast cancer survivor who reveals poor self-image and body integration during recovery from surgery. Nell is participating in an 8-week Dalcroze Eurhythmics class of 16 people designed for cancer survivors and caregivers. Nell attends the once-a-week class with her best friend—neither is a musician. During the class, the facilitator leads the participants through a wide range of rhythmic and movement-based activities, from finding their personal tempos through walking, tapping, and improvising movements; to developing a vocabulary of movement skills that allows them to express the rhythmic and musical elements of the music being played; and to solving musical problems with a partner in the class—demonstrating how the music can be expressed in motion. Every class culminates in a musical presentation— *plastique animée*—that allows participants to integrate the brain and the body in order to create a group movement improvisation that speaks to the elements of music and human feelings. Nell is asked to keep a journal on the experience and share the experience with the facilitator on a regular basis.

Conclusion

Music therapy has a valuable benefactor in Émile Jaques-Dalcroze. He believed that all people can and should experience music through singing, playing, listening, analyzing, improvising, and composing, regardless of ability. Some of his early work was with children with visual impairments, teaching them music as well as confidence and orientation skills through music and movement activities. Music exists for all people as a joyful experience. Through the integration of the physical, emotional, and intellectual powers of music, people may come to understand themselves better as well as those around them. Jaques-Dalcroze created a life that combined all that he loved: people, music, movement, drama, freedom, and a true zest for life—a precious legacy indeed.

References

Abramson, R. M. (1980). Dalcroze-based improvisation. *Music Educators Journal, 66*(5), 62–68.

Abramson, R. M. (2001). The approach of Emile Jaques-Dalcroze. In L. Choksy, R. M. Abramson, A. E. Gillespie, & D. Woods (Eds.), *Teaching music in the twenty-first century.* Upper Saddle River, NJ: Prentice Hall.

Brick, R. M. (1973). Eurhythmics: One aspect of audition. *Volta Review, 75*(3), 155–160.

Caldwell, J. T. (1993). A Dalcroze perspective on skills for learning music. *Music Educators Journal, 79*(7), 27–28.

Caldwell, J. T. (1995). *Expressive singing: Dalcroze Eurhythmics for voice.* Englewood Cliffs, NJ: Prentice Hall.

Campbell, P. S. (1991). Rhythmic movement and public school education: Progressive views in the formative years. *Journal of Research in Music Education, 19,* 12–22.

Carder, P. (Ed.). (1990). *The eclectic curriculum in American music education* (2nd ed.). Reston, VA: Music Educators National Conference.

Collins, D. L. (1993). *Teaching choral music.* Englewood Cliffs, NJ: Prentice Hall.

Dutoit, C. L. (1971). *Music movement therapy.* Geneva, Switzerland: Institut Jaques-Dalcroze.

Frego, R. J. D. (1995). Music movement therapy for people with AIDS: The use of music movement therapy as a form of palliative care for people with AIDS. *International Journal of Arts Medicine, 4*(2), 21–25.

Frego, R. J. D. (2007). Dalcroze Eurhythmics as a therapeutic tool. *The Canadian Dalcroze Society Journal/Bulletin de la Société Dalcroze du Canada, 1*(2), 3–4.

Gaston, E. T. (Ed.). (1968). *Music and therapy.* New York: Macmillan.

Gauger, L. A. (1995). *An investigation of the effect of rhythmic movement on patients with chronic schizophrenia.* Unpublished master's thesis, Texas Women's University, Denton.

Hibben, J. K. (1984). Movement as musical expression in a music therapy setting. *Music Therapy, 4,* 91–97.

Hibben, J. K. (1991). Identifying dimensions of music therapy activities appropriate for children at different stages of group development, *Arts in Psychotherapy, 18,* 301–310.

Johnson, M. D. (1993). Dalcroze skills for all teachers. *Music Educators Journal, 79*(8), 42–45.

Martin, F., Dénes, T., Berchtold, A., Gagnebin, H., Reichel, B., Dutoit, C., & Stadler, E. (1965). *Émile Jaques-Dalcroze: L'homme, le compositeur, le créateur de la rhythmique.* Neuchâtel, Swisse: Baconnière.

Mead, V. H. (1994). *Dalcroze eurhythmics in today's music classroom.* New York: Schott Music.

Minder-Jeanneret, I. (1995). Femmes musiciennes en Suisse romande: La musicienne professionnelle au tournant du siècle dans le miroir de la presse (1894–1914). *Collection Archives Vivantes.* Yens S./Morges [Suisse]: Editions Cabédita.

Odom, S. L. (1998). Jaques-Dalcroze, Emile. *International Encyclopedia of Dance, Vol. 3.* New York: Oxford.

Pennington, J. (1925). *The importance of being rhythmic.* New York: Knickerbocker Press.

Spector, I. (1990). *Rhythm and life: The work of Emile Jaques-Dalcroze.* Stuyvesant, NY: Pendragon Press.

Swaiko, N. (1974). The role and value of a eurhythmics program in a curriculum for deaf children. *American Annals of the Deaf, 119*(3), 155–160.

Recommended Additional Readings

Aronoff, F. W. (1983). Dalcroze strategies for music learning in the classroom. *International Journal of Music Education, 2,* 23–25.

Bachmann, M. L. (1991). *Dalcroze today. An education through and into music* (D. Parlett, Trans.). New York: Oxford University Press.

Brown, J., Sherrill, C., & Gench, B. (1981). Effects of an integrated physical education/music program in changing early childhood perceptual/motor performance. *Perceptual and Motor Skills, 53*(1), 151–154.

Driver, E. (1951). *A pathway to Dalcroze Eurhythmics.* London: T. Nelson and Sons.

Findlay, E. (1971). *Rhythm and movement: Applications of Dalcroze Eurhythmics.* Secaucus, NJ: Summy Birchard.

Frego, R. J. D., & Leck, H. (2005). *Creating artistry through movement* [DVD]. Milwaukee, WI: Hal Leonard.

Jaques-Dalcroze, E. (1920). *The Jaques-Dalcroze method of eurhythmics: Rhythmic movement* (Vols. 1 & 2). London: Novello. (Original work published 1918)

Jaques-Dalcroze, E. (1921). *Rhythm, music and education* (H. F. Rubinstein, Trans.). New York: G. P. Putnam's Sons. (Original work published 1921)

Jaques-Dalcroze, E. (1931). *Eurhythmics, art and education* (F. Rothwell, Trans.; C. Cox, Ed.). New York: Barnes. (Original work published 1930)

Joseph, A. (1982). *A Dalcroze Eurhythmics approach to music learning in kindergarten through rhythmic movement, ear-training and improvisation.* Doctoral dissertation, Carnegie Mellon University, Pittsburgh.

Schnebly-Black, J., & Moore, S. F. (1997). *The rhythm inside: connecting body, mind, and spirit through music.* Portland, OR: Rudra Press.

Chapter 4

The Kodály Approach to Music Therapy

Mike D. Brownell
R. J. David Frego
Eum-Mi Kwak
Amanda M. Rayburn

Introduction

Zoltán Kodály (1882–1960), Hungarian composer, musicologist, and music educator, played a pivotal role in the development of the Hungarian music education tradition and later of music education in the United States. To this day, Hungary has a rich musical culture. There are numerous orchestras and concert choirs throughout the country and significant emphasis is placed on music education. Beginning in childcare centers, music is part of the regular educational curriculum. Kodály was born in Kecskemét, Hungary. His family then moved to Galánta, a small town in western Hungary (now Slovakia) where Kodály spent 7 years of his childhood (Ledbetter, 1996). During his childhood and young adulthood, he explored many different genres of music and developed a musical preference and enthusiasm for Hungarian folk music. Even though his parents were not professional musicians, his father played violin and his mother had a fine voice. Often, family friends would bring their instruments to Kodály's home and, together with his parents, form a small chamber ensemble. As a result, Kodály was exposed to chamber folk music at an early age. In addition, he had several opportunities to listen to the children of the famous Miók's gypsy band, since they performed in the same area where Kodály grew up.

After moving to Nagyszonmbat in 1892, Kodály began studying the piano, violin, and cello. He mastered all three instruments within a few years and joined the orchestra and choir of the local cathedral. In 1905, Kodály began to collect and analyze Hungarian and other folk music with his friend and fellow Hungarian composer, Béla Bartók. On their first expedition together, they collected more than 150 folk songs. These works were analyzed and classified according to mode and scale and eventually became the first volume of the massive *Corpus Musicae Popularis Hungaricae* (Hungarian Folk Music). It is a collaboration that includes 12 volumes containing 2,700 Magyar folk songs, 3,500 Magyar-Romanian folk songs, and several hundred Turkish and North African folk songs (Eosze, 1962).

Kodály was a prolific composer, and many of his works belong to the realm of famous 20th-century compositions. Like Bartók, he based many of his works on the folk idioms of Hungary. While avidly composing, Kodály traveled to various villages and towns collecting and recording folk songs and tune variants. His collective activity stimulated his work on music education. Kodály became one of the greatest proponents of music education in the 20th century. He placed tremendous value on and stressed the importance of quality music education:

> It is much more important who is the music teacher in Kisvárda than who is the director of the opera house in Budapest . . . for a poor director fails once, but a poor teacher keeps on failing for thirty years, killing the love of music in thirty batches of children. (Choksy, 1988, p. 3)

The composer focused his attention on music education in 1925 and actively began to formulate the basic principles of the Kodály philosophy. Kodály believed that (a) music should belong to everyone; (b) children should learn their musical "mother tongue" first, like they learn their linguistic mother tongue; and (c) children should receive training in singing, reading, and notating music during the early years of formal education (Carder, 1990; Choksy, 1988). Kodály's beliefs and ensuing work were extended and developed by his disciples and followers in Hungary and countries abroad.

During the 1960s, music educators throughout the world began learning about the Kodály approach as a result of presentations at the International Society for Music Education (ISME) conferences. Music educators from eastern and western Europe, Japan, Australia, New Zealand, North and South America, South Africa, and Iceland visited Hungary, learned the Kodály approach, and subsequently began to implement it in their own countries. In the United States, the approach began to gain momentum at the ISME conference at Interlochen, Michigan, and the Kodály Method symposium at Stanford University in 1966 (Choksy, 1988).

The Approach

Theory and Principles

Kodály emphasized that music training begins early in life with the teaching and learning of music through direct experiences and encounters. In Kodály's words, "Often a single experience will open the young soul to music for a whole lifetime. This experience cannot be left to chance; it is the duty of the school to provide it" (Organization of American Kodály Educators [OAKE], 1965). Observing the poor quality of musicianship and the illiteracy among the people in his native Hungary, Kodály envisioned achieving one essential goal: music literacy (Shehan, 1986). Kodály asked, "Is it imaginable that anybody who is unable to read words can acquire a literary culture or knowledge of any kind? Equally, no musical knowledge of any kind can be acquired without the reading of music" (Hoffer, 1993, p. 125). Systematic teaching and training of musical skills included reading, writing, and listening to shape the development of music literacy. Kodály said, "Teach music and singing at school in such a way that it is not a torture but a joy for the pupil; instill a thirst for finer music in him, a thirst which will last for a lifetime" (OAKE, 1965). Kodály aspired to make music more accessible to people, and he served as a pioneer for elevating the standards of music education (Shehan, 1986). One of the objectives of the approach is to assist in "the well-balanced social and artistic development of the child" (Choksy, 1999) and to develop the "complete musician" (OAKE, 1965).

Key Elements of the Approach

The Kodály approach is based on four key elements: singing, folk music, solfège, and the movable *do*. Kodály believed that the first key element, singing, was essential to teach, learn, and understand music. Therefore, he claimed that the development of the natural singing voice is key because it allows for musical self-expression and trains the inner, musical ear (OAKE, 1965). Kodály primarily taught by singing a cappella, stating that "Only the human voice, which is a possession of everyone, and at the same time the most beautiful of all instruments, can serve as the basis for a general music culture" (Hoffer, 1993, p. 127). Through singing, a person produces his or her own unique sound that facilitates the learning process and creates a stronger sense of accomplishment and fulfillment (OAKE, 1965).

The second key element of the Kodály approach is the use of folk music. Kodály exposed his students to what he considered the best music resources, including authentic folk music, children's songs and games, and pedagogical exercises by recognized composers (Choksy, 1999; Hoffer, 1993; OAKE, 1965). Most of Kodály's pedagogical approach, developed after World War II, focuses on Hungarian folk songs. The Nationalistic movement clearly influenced Kodály and the native people of Hungary. The people of his country sought to preserve their own music and language to maintain their national identity and roots. Kodály expressed his views on the value of folk music:

> Folk songs offer such a rich variety of moods and perspective, that the child grows in human consciousness and feels more and more at home in his country. . . . To become international we first have to belong to one distinct people and to speak its language properly, not in gibberish. To understand other people, we must first understand ourselves. And nothing will accomplish this better than a thorough knowledge of one's native folk songs. (Hoffer, 1993, p. 128)

The third and fourth key elements, solfège and movable *do* are two techniques that Kodály's approach employs to develop pitch awareness and auditory discrimination. The movable *do* system, an English choral training technique, represents relative pitch, and solfège represents fixed pitch. Solfège, however, facilitates the skill of inner hearing where the child can reproduce a pitch in his or her mind without singing the pitch aloud. The hand signals developed by John Curwen were also adapted for use in this approach. Each hand sign corresponds to a pitch syllable. Hand signs serve as a visual representation of the space and relationship among notes that facilitates interval reading and vocal sight singing. The hand is adjusted according to how high and low the notes are and the size of the interval sung. Musical shorthand, the first letter of the solfège syllable, is used when writing the solfège with the stem notation to make writing and musical dictation easier and quicker. After understanding the concept of hand signs, children apply them to folk music that uses the pentatonic scale (Choksy, 1999; Hoffer, 1993).

Using pentatonic music extensively at the initial stages of musical development enables the child to feel more comfortable when introduced to major and minor modes. The tonic note or tonal center of a song is *do* in a major mode, and the sixth scale degree, *la*, becomes the tonal center in a song in a minor mode. The minor third between *sol* and *mi* is usually the first interval that children are taught. The minor third sounds the same regardless of the mode of the song; therefore, the child is able to learn the placement of these notes on a staff. After mastery of this intervalic relationship, other notes and intervals that make up the pentatonic scale may follow (Hoffer, 1993; OAKE, 1965; Shehan, 1986; Szonyi, 1973).

In addition to the four key elements, the Kodály approach uses another technique called *solmization*. It consists of syllables that represent note durations. Stick or stem notation is used in conjunction with these syllables. The rhythmic syllable is often said to the value or duration of the note. For example, the quarter note is "ta" (♩); the eighth note is "ti-ti" (♫); the sixteenth note is "ti-ri-ti-ri" (♬♬); the half note is "ta-a" (♩); the dotted half note is "ta-a-a" (♩); the whole note is "ta-a-a-a" (o). Rhythm is first presented through iconic picture cards that represent the notes; each picture adjusts in size to the duration of the note. After further practice of these rhythm syllables, music flash cards with stick notation can be made to help children with their visual tracking skills and the speed and accuracy of reading rhythms (Choksy, 1999; Hoffer, 1993; Strong, 1983).

Sequence of the Approach

Kodály's approach can best be described as a child developmental approach rather than a subject-logic approach to teaching. The subject-logic approach focuses not on the child but on musical content. For example, rhythm is taught using what would appear to be the most logical and reasonable way, with the whole note presented first and then the half note. Kodály's approach, being a child developmental approach, begins with moving rhythms, such as quarter and eighth notes, instead of the sustained note used in the subject-logic approach. This facilitates the child being able to use movement in conjunction with rhythm learning. The sequential approach begins with the child's natural abilities and with what the child can learn most easily (Szonyi, 1973).

The success of Kodály's teaching approach is due to the carefully planned, sequential presentation of musical concepts and the direct experiences that occur. Kodály states:

> Music must not be approached from its intellectual, rational side, nor should it be conveyed to the child as a system of algebraic symbols, or as a secret writing of a language to which he has no connection. The way should be paved for direct intuition. (OAKE, 1965)

Curriculum

In order to love music, Kodály believed that a deep knowledge and understanding of music must be obtained. The presentation of materials, concepts, and development of skills will be more meaningful to the learner if the curriculum is revealed one step at a time through a sequential process, using the concept of "sound before symbol." The four stages that must be applied to Kodály's approach include the following:

Prepare: The teacher prepares the child for new material through new songs that contain the new material to be learned. The teacher actively engages the child through musical activities, allowing the child to experience the new material firsthand. The musical activities include rote singing, singing loudly or softly, clapping the rhythm, stepping to the beat, singing faster or slower, and playing singing games. This stage is complete after learning a core of songs.

Make Conscious: The teacher provides a musical opportunity for conscious awareness of a new concept through one particular song. The children are asked specific questions to promote discovery of the new musical element of rhythm or melody. When the questions are answered, the teacher identifies the new element and presents it either through hand signs, showing the new rhythm, or notating the element on a staff.

Reinforce: In the reinforcement stage, the teacher reverts to some of the techniques in the first stage. The new element is identified in each of the songs learned during the preparation stage and the children are now reading from notation, using rhythm syllables and solfège. In addition, the children may even notate certain phrases of the song that contain the new element. They are exposed to more music to practice using the new element.

Assess: The last stage allows the child to read new songs with the melodic or rhythmic elements so that the element is internalized and remembered. The child applies or generalizes the new melodic turn or rhythmic motive to other situations or musical activities that include improvisation and composition. Each of the four stages is repeated for each of the new rhythmic and melodic elements to be learned. For each melodic turn learned, the teacher overlaps by preparing a new rhythmic element. This learning process provides the opportunity for material to be ingrained in the mind, thereby allowing the student to acquire a deeper knowledge of music (Boshkoff, 1991; Choksy, 1999).

When selecting songs to teach musical skills and concepts, the teacher must first consider the frequency with which the melodic or rhythmic pattern occurs and its position in the song. Songs should contain the musical element to be learned in the first phrase of the song rather than in the middle or at the end. Repetition of the new element throughout the song is another consideration. Furthermore, songs selected for learning purposes should be simple and repetitive to facilitate ease of learning.

Kodály's curriculum provides sequenced steps of musical behaviors from the elementary level to the secondary level. The progress made is affected by three main factors: (a) the frequency and length of music lessons, (b) the previous musical experiences of the children, and (c) the comfort level and competence of the teacher using the Kodály techniques. When developing a sequential lesson plan, the teacher must consider the students to whom the lesson will be given. Lesson planning using the Kodály approach requires both structure and flexibility for the teaching/learning process to be successful (Boshkoff, 1991; Choksy, 1999; OAKE, 1965).

Implications for Programs in North America

Kodály's approach is being used more frequently with elementary school students than secondary school students. One reason that teachers in secondary schools do not use the Kodály approach may be lack of familiarity with the approach, or that curriculum is performance-oriented rather than focused on teaching musical rudiments. Kodály's approach, however, is adaptable and can be used at all levels of music education in North American schools (Turpin, 1986).

At the elementary level, the Kodály approach is taught in frequent, short sessions. The program uses movement and singing activities that teach musical concepts through exploration and discovery. Several musical principles that the approach employs include the following concepts: (a) loud and soft, (b) fast and slow, (c) same and different (form), (d) simple versus compound duple meter, (e) melody, (f) short and long (rhythm), and (g) timbre (Choksy, 1999).

Similarly, the approach can also be applied effectively to secondary choral and instrumental music in North American schools. In secondary music programs, the desired outcome must first be addressed in order to determine specific objectives and to identify instructional strategies to achieve musical goals. Choral music teachers may use hand signs to rehearse songs that are in different modes and that contain difficult intervals. Furthermore, the teacher can present a tune through the use of Curwen hand signs and have the students identify the song through the concept of inner hearing. Likewise, the instrumental teacher can use warm-up exercises to develop independence on the student's instrument part by having the student use hand signs while simultaneously singing the notes in solfège. Challenging rhythmic patterns can be learned by having the student isolate measures that contain the difficult rhythms, and the student must speak the rhythmic syllables while clapping the correct note values (Choksy, 1999; Turpin, 1986).

Music Therapy Applications

The greatest tenet of Kodály's philosophy is that music should be made available to all children. Five general principles and objectives contribute to this belief:

1. The innate musicality present in all children should be developed to the fullest extent possible.
2. The language of music should be made known to children in the same way as spoken language so that they might be able to read, write, and create with the vocabulary of music.
3. Folk songs and musical heritage should be passed down to children.
4. The great music of the world should be made available and accessible to all children.
5. Music is necessary for human development and should not be thought of as a triviality. (Bonis, 1964; Choksy, Abramson, Gillespie, & Woods, 1986; Williams, 1975)

Kodály made these statements regarding music education, yet many of them clearly apply to the field of music therapy. Kodály's principal belief that music should be made available for everyone closely parallels Gaston's (1968) belief that "all mankind has need for aesthetic expression and experience" (p. 21). This philosophy is especially important as it applies to music therapists in school settings, who may need to adapt the music curriculum for children with disabilities. Additionally, therapists working privately can incorporate these techniques when providing adapted musical lessons to individuals with disabilities. The principles and techniques of this approach are most aptly applied to special education. Strong (1983) notes that "Although

Kodály may never have spoken directly concerning special education, the Kodály Approach may be the best means of achieving his ambitious goal of music belonging to everyone by making music literacy accessible to the exceptional child" (p. 3).

The developmental approach of the Kodály approach may be the quality that is most essential to provide security and successful experiences for children with disabilities. Intellectual understanding of music is not considered until the child is physically capable of performing the music (Lathom, 1974). This approach is also based on multisensory experiences. The Curwen hand signs offer a physical representation of the notes being sung and offer an additional mode of sensory input (Lathom, 1974). Visual aids may help individuals with disabilities learn various musical and nonmusical skills. For example, hand signals, a felt board, and pictures to represent words can provide a visual representation of the material to be learned. These visual aids serve as an extrasensory modality and iconic representation in the therapy session. Music education, both for individuals with disabilities and typically developing peers, serves to benefit from the combination of as many different multimodal strategies as possible (Gault, 2005). Speaking of the application of the Kodály approach in special education, Strong (1983) states:

> Since one of the normal avenues of learning may be blocked or malfunctioning in the mind of the exceptional child, the fact that each music concept can be presented through visual, aural, and kinesthetic senses makes musical learning through the Kodály Approach that much more accessible to the exceptional child. The approach is based on task analysis and successive approximations. Each step must be comfortable for the child before moving on to the next task. Kodály stressed the importance of repetition and the simplistic nature of the music to enhance the learning process. When working with students with various learning disabilities or with mental retardation, the therapist must allow for repetition of the music so that ample opportunity for the student to elicit the appropriate behavior or response is allowed. The music therapist also sequences the music similar to the task involved in therapy to provide successful experiences for the exceptional child. The sequenced, predictable music thus facilitates the student's feelings of security and comfort. Because the approach focuses on quality of outcome rather than quantity, the speed at which materials are presented is easily adapted to fit the learning styles of each individual student or class. (p. 4)

Kodály set out to educate the children of his native Hungary under the premise that music should be made available to all people. This principle, along with the techniques of the approach itself, has been adopted by music educators all over the world (Choksy, 1999; Eosze, 1962). Music therapists may also adopt the fluidity and adaptability of the Kodály approach and incorporate it in their clinical practice.

Also of note to music therapists are the potential nonmusical domains for which elements of the Kodály approach may be applicable. Research in this area has focused primarily on typically developing populations; Kodály-based education has been shown to improve perceptual-motor development (Brown, Sherril, & Gency, 1981; Gromko & Poorman, 1998; Kalmar, 1982); increase temporal and spatial abilities (Hanson, 2003; Hurwitz, Wolff, Bortnick, & Kokas, 1975); facilitate the acquisition of language and social skills (Gan & Chong, 1998); and even produce positive effects on general intelligence (Hurwitz et al., 1975; Laczo, 1985). Additional research utilizing subjects with disabilities is still needed to empirically demonstrate the usefulness of these techniques to music therapists when applied judiciously.

Examples of Music Therapy Applications

Brenda is an 8-year-old girl with spastic cerebral palsy who exhibits deficits in her language skills. Dan, a board-certified music therapist, designed an intervention that uses the Kodály approach to address the acquisition of expressive language skills. Brenda has difficulties expressing her thoughts in words, so she was asked to supply a word or phrase in the context of the song "Who's Got a Fishpole?" After she successfully completed this step, Brenda was asked to create a new verse for the song. A visual representation of the rhythms of phrases she created was presented, and the phrase was incorporated into the song. Brenda was asked to sing the phrases that she created using the rhythms provided by the music therapist. Dan supplemented subsequent sessions with other songs to which Brenda could add words or phrases. Through additional work on these songs, Dan further increased Brenda's language development by addressing areas such as inflection and articulation.

Peggy is a music therapist who works with children with special needs in a special education classroom in a public school. Peggy received some training in the Kodály approach and frequently incorporates these techniques into her sessions. An intervention was designed to increase gross motor skills. Peggy illustrates percussion patterns on the board using pictures of feet, hands, and legs; each of these pictures represents the body part to be used to produce the percussion. The intervention developed body awareness, balance, agility, and strength.

Alex is a 12-year-old male diagnosed with Asperger Syndrome who has displayed some emerging musical proclivities. Alex's mother has taken him to several local music teachers in an effort to capitalize on his interest but has run into difficulties locating an instructor who is able to accommodate her son's behavior difficulties and inability to follow along in a standard music method book. She was referred to a local music therapist who offered adapted music lessons. Using the tenets of the Kodály approach, the music therapist was able to tailor a piano curriculum ideally suited for Alex that functioned independently from the piano books with which he had struggled in the past. The "sound before symbol" concept was especially useful in helping Alex master such concepts as intervallic relationships and rhythm, long before they were introduced in written form, ensuring that Alex had command of the concept before being burdened by notation. The multisensory approach also held Alex's attention through the duration of his lessons.

David is a 9-year-old boy with a mild cognitive impairment in an inclusive general music classroom. The instructor is attempting to fully integrate David into the class but is having difficulties because David is unable to read rhythms at the same level as his typically achieving peers. The teacher employs the Kodály technique of rhythmic solemnization to teach the relationship between quarter and eighth notes. David was asked to walk in rhythm while the teacher said "ta," and to run in place when the teacher says "ti-ti." Once this skill was mastered, the teacher wrote the syllables on the board and asked David to repeat the walking/running exercise while she pointed to the syllables. Typical rhythmic notation was then superimposed over the syllables, and a hand drum was used in place of walking and running. The syllables were gradually phased out, and at this point David was able to visually distinguish between the two note values and was able to participate more fully with his classroom peers.

Conclusion

The Kodály approach is a versatile and adaptable approach that can be used to teach a variety of concepts, both musical and academic. The developmental and performance aspects of the approach make it appropriate for the music therapy clinical setting. The sequential teaching strategies used in Kodály-based lessons have important implications for shaping client behaviors. Kodály's stages of reinforcement and assessment are particularly applicable to music therapy clinical techniques. Moreover, all populations of music therapy clientele can benefit from a better understanding of music and improved musical skills by using this approach.

References

Bonis, F. (1964). *The selected writings of Zoltan Kodály* (L. Halapy & F. Macnicol, Trans.). London: Boosey & Hawkes.

Boshkoff, R. (1991). Lesson planning the Kodály way. *Music Educators Journal, 79,* 30–34.

Brown, J., Sherril, C., & Gency, B. (1981). Effects of an integrated physical education/music program in changing early childhood perceptual-motor performance. *Perceptual and Motor Skills, 53,* 151–154.

Carder, P. (1990). *The eclectic curriculum in American music education* (2nd ed.). Reston, VA: Music Educators National Conference.

Choksy, L. (1988). *The Kodály method: Comprehensive musical education from infant to adult* (2nd ed.). Englewood Cliffs, NJ: Prentice Hall.

Choksy, L. (1999). *The Kodály Method I–III.* Englewood Cliffs, NJ: Prentice Hall.

Choksy, L., Abramson, R., Gillespie, A., & Woods, D. (1986). *Teaching music in the twentieth century.* Englewood Cliffs, NJ: Prentice-Hall.

Eosze, L. (1962). *Zoltan Kodály: His life and work* (I. Farkas & G. Gulyas, Trans.). London: Collet's Holdings.

Gan, L., & Chong, S. (1998). The rhythm of language: Fostering oral and listening skills in Singapore preschool children through an integrated music and language arts program. *Early Child Development and Care, 144,* 39–45.

Gaston, E. T. (Ed.). (1968). *Music in therapy.* New York: Macmillan Press.

Gault, B. (2005). Music learning through all the channels: Combining aural, visual, and kinesthetic strategies to develop musical understanding. *General Music Today, 19,* 7–9.

Gromko, J. E., & Poorman, A. S. (1998). The effect of music training on preschoolers' spatial-temporal task performance. *Journal of Research in Music Education, 46,* 173–181.

Hanson, M. (2003). Effects of sequenced Kodaly literacy-based music instruction on the spatial reasoning skills of kindergarten students. *Research and Issues in Music Education.* Retrieved April 17, 2008, from http://www.stthomas.edu/rimeonline/vol1/hanson1.htm

Hoffer, C. (1993). *International curriculum developments: An introduction to music education* (2nd ed.). Belmont, CA: Wadsworth.

Hurwitz, I., Wolff, P. H., Bortnick, B. D., & Kokas, K. (1975). Nonmusical effects of the Kodaly music curriculum in primary grade children. *Journal of Learning Disabilities, 8,* 167–174.

Kalmar, M. (1982). The effects of music education based on Kodaly's directives in nursery school children; from a psychologist's point of view. *Psychology of Music, 1982 Special Issue*, 63–68.

Laczo, Z. (1985). The nonmusical outcomes of music education: Influence on intelligence. *Bulletin of the Council for Research in Music Education, 85,* 109–118.

Lathom, W. (1974). Application of Kodály concepts in music therapy. *Journal of Music Therapy, 11,* 13–20.

Ledbetter, S. (1996). *Zoltan Kodály (1882–1967).* Retrieved from http://www.proarte.org/notes/Kodály.htm

Organization of American Kodály Educators (OAKE). (1965). *The Kodály concept of music education* [Brochure]. New York: Boosey & Hawkes.

Shehan, P. (1986). Major approaches to music education: An account of method. *Music Educators Journal, 72,* 26–31.

Strong, A. D. (1983). The Kodály method applied to special education. *Kodály Envoy, 9*(3), 3–8.

Szonyi, E. (1973). *Kodály's principles in practice: An approach to music education through the Kodály method.* New York: Boosey & Hawkes.

Turpin, D. (1986). Kodály, Dalcroze, Orff, and Suzuki: Application in the secondary schools. *Music Educators Journal, 72,* 56–59.

Williams, M. (1975). Philosophical foundations of the Kodály approach to education. *Kodály Envoy, 2*(2), 4–9.

Recommended Additional Readings

Nash, G. C. (1974). *Creative approaches to child development with music, language, and movement: Incorporating the philosophies and techniques of Orff, Kodály and Laban.* Los Angeles: Alfred.

Zemke, L. (1976). *Kodály: 35 lesson plans and folk song supplement.* Champaign, IL: Mark Foster Music.

Psychotherapeutic Approaches
to Music Therapy

Chapter 5

The Bonny Method of Guided Imagery and Music

Debra Burns
Jennifer Woolrich

Introduction

The Bonny Method of Guided Imagery and Music (BMGIM) is a "music-centered exploration of consciousness, which uses specifically sequenced classical music programs to stimulate and sustain a dynamic unfolding of inner experiences" (Association for Music and Imagery [AMI], 2008b). BMGIM practitioners contend that (a) both imagery and music are therapeutic agents; (b) the therapeutic process includes cognitive, psychodynamic, and transpersonal aspects; and (c) expanded awareness results in major therapeutic benefits. Therapists work with a variety of populations, including clients adjusting to chronic illness or seeking personal and spiritual growth. At present, there are over 100 BMGIM therapists in the United States. Training programs exist in the United States, Europe, Australia, New Zealand, and Japan.

Music provides a basis for self-expression; in addition, it provides organization of the self (Ruud, 1980). In light of this, BMGIM is based on the humanistic and transpersonal theories that emphasize the awareness of the individual and the influence of music on ego development. Classical music in BMGIM assists in achieving therapeutic goals by helping the client concentrate and consequently become more absorbed in his or her internal experience. Music provides structure and direction for the experience, facilitates emotional expression, and contributes to peak experiences (Bonny & Pahnke, 1972).

Music acts as a stimulus that releases unconscious material for therapeutic use. Unconscious material can include images, feelings, and thoughts associated with the client's present and past experiences. Musical elements such as form, dynamics, timbre, and rhythm provide a predictable structure that in turn gives the client a sense of security. This predictability and security encourages the client to confront emotionally laden unconscious material. Confrontation with unconscious conflicts facilitates the release of emotions and contributes to psychological understanding and subsequent behavioral change.

History and Development

Inspired by a peak experience while playing the violin, Helen Bonny used music in combination with relaxation to facilitate similar client experiences at the Maryland Psychiatric Research Center. BMGIM was developed as a result of research on the use of LSD to enhance patients' therapy (Bonny & Savary, 1990). The researchers attempted to elicit peak experiences, using LSD as a method to transcend the limitations of consciousness. Eventually, music was also integrated into the therapy sessions and the benefits of music were quickly noticed. The music was able to narrow the patients' attention and heighten their concentration, which allowed them to focus more on the experience.

As the government began to cut funding for LSD research, music became the focus of experimental investigation. Researchers began to investigate whether music alone could guide a patient to a peak experience. The data indicated that music did indeed lead patients to a deeper level of consciousness, and hence facilitate peak experiences. By 1974, BMGIM listening programs were developed and structured sessions were based on these musical programs.

Humanistic and Transpersonal Theories in Relation to the Bonny Method

BMGIM is based on humanistic and transpersonal psychologies that aim to increase self-awareness and understanding. The origins of humanistic psychology are based primarily on the writings of Abraham Maslow. Maslow developed a theory of motivation whereby an individual progresses from basic physiological needs to the complex needs that he called self-actualization. Self-actualization is a self-initiated drive to reach one's greatest human potential. Humanistic psychotherapy seeks to help the individual progress through these stages (Maslow, 1968). Listening to music in altered states of consciousness may elicit insightful peak experiences that assist a person in reaching self-actualization (AMI, 2008a).

The purpose of transpersonal psychology, an extension of humanistic psychology, is for the client to acquire an expanded awareness of the self. The initial experiences within transpersonal therapy sessions encourage clients to fulfill basic needs as well as emotional, mental, and spiritual needs. By meeting all of their needs, clients are able to understand the self as a whole and to reach their optimal level of identity and obtain self-actualization. Therapeutic experiences encourage the client to travel inward and gain a better understanding of his or her inner world and increase one's sense of identity to include transpersonal dimensions of being. The inner search leads to a wisdom that enables the client to move toward wholeness and transcendence (Vaughan, 1979).

One of the main goals of transpersonal psychology is to encourage clients to tap into their own internal resources. Transpersonal psychologists believe that all clients have the potential to grow and develop independently by following a natural course of personal healing. The therapist does not solve clients' problems, but supports clients as they gain knowledge through insights that occur during therapy. Through transpersonal therapy, clients are able to go beyond the limitations of awareness at the ego level and experience a more complete self-understanding through imagery and dreams. These images include mythical, archetypal, and symbolic realms of inner experience. Through these images, clients experience a realization of self. Clients are able to view their identity as separate parts and resolve any internal conflicts. Clients then progress through a reintegration process and transcend ego boundaries (Vaughan, 1979).

The ultimate goal of the experiences in transpersonal psychology is self-transcendence. This occurs when clients understand themselves not "as totally isolated, but as part of something larger, inherently connected, and related to everything" (Vaughan, 1979). Clients understand how they fit into a universe intertwined through relationships. Clients must then accept their own purpose and responsibility in this universe. Once clients achieve a full understanding of themselves and the universe, they gain a sense of personal freedom, inner direction, and responsibility (Vaughan, 1979).

Abrams (2002) synthesizes the work of transpersonal psychologists and BMGIM practitioners to craft a specific transpersonal BMGIM theory to explain transpersonal phenomenon as it occurs within BMGIM sessions. This theory explains the interaction between the four elements of BMGIM sessions (music program listening, imagery, consciousness, and guide) with each other and within their totality, along with the process during which transpersonal experiences occur. An understanding of how transpersonal experiences occur within a BMGIM session allows the guide (therapist) to determine the best interventions within the session in order to deepen the experience.

The Function of the Music

The function of the music in BMGIM is to facilitate the imagery experience. Results from research suggest that music may enhance imagery by making the images more vivid (McKinney, 1990; McKinney & Tims, 1995; Peach, 1984; Quittner & Glueckauf, 1983) and providing structure and control during the imagery experience (Burns, 2000). However, the music must suggest the appropriate type of imagery given the client's individual needs and goals. Bonny (1972) developed a series of listening programs that contained emotional characteristics based on the melodic contour, dynamic range, harmonic structure, rhythm, and orchestration of the music. The names of these programs suggest the emotional characteristics that the music portrays: Comforting, Positive Affect, Affect Release, Imagery, and so forth (Bonny, 1978b). These programs are standard music for use with BMGIM therapy.

Therapists' choice of music is central to the therapeutic environment in that the music structures the imagery experience. The therapist demonstrates an understanding of the client's needs by choosing appropriate music. Historically, music has been chosen based on the iso-principle. This principle suggests that the selected piece of music should match the prevailing mood of the client. To make a music selection, the therapist must decide what mood the music portrays as well as discern the client's prevailing mood. Thus, to choose appropriate music for the client, the therapist must interpret and mirror the client's internal struggle and choose music that mirrors the struggle. By doing so, the therapist's projections and transferences may enter into the therapeutic environment, and the music may not provide adequate structure for the client's imagery experience.

Summer (1993) introduced the idea of choosing music based on Winnicott's Good Enough Mothering principle. With this principle, choosing music that is too relaxing and has clear structure with little variability does not challenge the client to move beyond the area of emotional comfort. Change within the client is encouraged if the music has some structural ambiguity that raises anxiety and encourages imagery. However, music that has little structure may provoke too much anxiety for the client. Summer likens the Good Enough Mothering principle to the analogy of a small child exploring his environment and then returning to his mother's arms. Similarly, music can be conceptualized as a container for the imagery experience. The size of the container is dictated by the level of arousal or anxiety that the client is experiencing. High levels of arousal require music that is more structured and predictable (smaller container), providing an opportunity to reduce arousal and focus attention on the imagery experience. Music that is less structured and unpredictable creates additional anxiety, hampering the client's ability to engage in the imagery experience. Once again, the size of container, or predictability of the music, is dependent on the goals and objectives of the BMGIM session.

The Function of Imagery and Emotion

Imagery that represents internal struggles elicits many types of emotional responses. Goldberg (1992) presented a Field Theory Model of BMGIM positing that the emotional content within a BMGIM session results from arousal of autonomic nervous system. This arousal of emotion leads to image formation. As the affective content of the music changes, the emotional arousal varies and influences the movement of the imagery. Stimulation of the nervous system begins with the auditory nerve that delivers musical stimuli from the ear into the cochlear nuclei up into the inferior colliculus and eventually through the reticular formation. The reticular formation extends through most of the brain stem up into the thalamus and eventually the hypothalamus. The hypothalamus is one neuroanatomical structure that makes up the limbic system and is involved in immune response. Little is known about the role of the limbic system in music processing, although one could postulate that perceptions of mood while listening to a piece of music might be processed within this system.

As the music arouses the neuroanatomical structures, it may trigger emotions that are predominant in the client. These emotions may be unconscious or conscious. If the client is unaware of the emotion, unable to tolerate it, or both, the image will appear as a representation of the emotion (Goldberg, 1992). During this process, the music is always in the environment and recedes from awareness as the client becomes increasingly immersed in the imagery. As the imagery recedes, the client becomes increasingly aware of the music again. If the music does not support the image, the emotional expression may be lost. As the client's emotions evolve, so do the client's images.

Physiological activation does not become an emotional experience until the client interprets the arousal. If clients find the arousal too threatening, they may engage in what Goldberg (1992) terms "a defensive maneuver" (p. 12). She reasons that this process may explain the emotionally laden images that are unaccompanied by affect or incongruent with the image. The purpose of the defensive maneuver is to decrease the amount of threat or stress that the client perceives "by deflecting, changing, or repressing the emotional response to music and the issue it represents" (p. 12). Defensive maneuvers may appear as the suppression of emotion, images, or personal issues. Emotional suppression may be characterized by client complaints that the music is bothersome. Cartoon images may represent an attempt to lessen the impact of the original image. Defensive maneuvers of personal issues may be evident if the imagery is disconnected.

Goldberg (1995) provides an example of her emotion theory that includes a defensive maneuver. She describes a 21-year-old male, hospitalized after an overdose of antidepressant medication. The patient was unable to rationalize any reason for his depression. Here is a description of the music/imagery portion of his first session:

> I'm lying under a tree, relaxing. There's a river, flowers. My friend is here. Men are running, running toward me. They're on the other side of the river. I feel uptight. I'm in a park now, with my dog. I'm a little boy. There's my father. He's asking where my dog is. I'm just staring at him. (p. 125)

The patient ended the session prematurely because he could not tolerate the image of his father. Evidently, his father had died before the client's birthday a couple of years earlier and the family dynamics were such that he was not allowed to express his grief. The client "vulnerability was evident in his inability to suppress or transform overwhelming affect and images through defensive maneuvers" (p. 126).

The ability of the client to form defensive maneuvers may suggest the development of ego strength or coping strategies. In addition, emotionally laden issues may become apparent with the onset of defensive maneuvers. Goldberg explains that the healthy client can keep anxiety at a manageable level and quickly move through defensive maneuvers during the session. In contrast, unhealthy clients are less likely to form defensive maneuvers and become emotionally overwhelmed. The therapist assessment of defensive maneuvers dictates how much support and structure the client requires.

Through the BMGIM process, clients learn to take control of their imagery experiences and work with the music to elicit positive feelings and eventually greater self-worth. This process requires the client to experience emotions associated with images that occur during the music listening portion of the session. As the mood of the person improves, the images evoked during therapy sessions should reflect this transformation.

Rinker (1991) describes the transformation of a client's imagery from desolate to nurturing. The client's first image was that of hot sand in her throat. The client decided that this image was related to her family's message not to talk about feelings and conflicts. Therefore, any time the client felt like expressing herself, the image of hot sand in her throat appeared, thus symbolizing her emotional inhibition. Working through this conflict, the client's imagery began to change as she became more self-aware and continued to use her painful emotional experiences as a child to grow. During a pivotal session, the client began crying, and her tears were imaged as "golden tears surrounded by a rainbow of blues and purples" (p. 314). These tears washed away her pain as an additional image of the rising sun appeared. The therapist observed a moment of silence in the client before a beautiful smile appeared on her face. The client reported being in the sunlight and thinking that all she had done was good.

In 2002, Goldberg expanded her Field Theory Model to the Holographic Model to more fully include the various states of consciousness experienced during a BMGIM session, the role of the Self, and psychospiritual growth and processes (Goldberg, 2002). According to Webster's dictionary, a hologram is a three-dimensional image created from a reflected light interfering with a reference beam (Landau, 2003). Within Goldberg's holographic field there is music, the music-emotion-imagery cycle, the Self, and various states of consciousness (Goldberg, 2002). Visually, the holograph allows for a multitude of music-emotion-imagery cycles, or multiple therapeutic processes occurring simultaneously. Additionally, the holograph allows for additional levels of consciousness including, but not limited to, biographic information (memory), ego, and persona. These levels of consciousness also include areas of expanded awareness, including transcendental and transpersonal experiences.

Another aspect of the Holographic Model involves the role of the Self, which Goldberg conceptualizes as all areas of consciousness, known and unknown. The music within a BMGIM session assists the Self in discovering those areas of consciousness that are unknown and are yet to be integrated. The process of psychospiritual growth within BMGIM can be described as the integration of consciousness, with ego development and spiritual growth occurring simultaneously (Goldberg, 2002).

Characteristics of the Therapist

The role of the therapist is one of support and encouragement. He or she must empathize with the client while at the same time provide the therapeutic structure the client needs to progress through the therapeutic process. Bonny (1978a) identified three qualifications of a guide that lend themselves to successful therapeutic practice in Guided Imagery and Music: personality, training, and commitment. Therapists need to be able to allow and give permission for the client to lead the session. Also important is the therapist's ability to allow the client to experience intense affective responses. The BMGIM therapist must be aware of the theoretical underpinnings of responses to musical stimuli. Therapists must also have a thorough knowledge of music history, theory, and psychoacoustics.

Knowledge of therapeutic techniques, altered states of consciousness, dream analysis, and psychopathology also helps the BMGIM therapist be effective in working with clients. Bonny (1978a) contends that dedication and commitment are also essential in working with BMGIM clients. These two elements are important because those who practice BMGIM must believe in BMGIM's effectiveness in encouraging self-healing. Although these qualities are important for a therapist, over involvement may cloud the therapist's judgment and not allow the discernment needed to assess clients' progress. Overinvolvement in the BMGIM process may also bias the therapist enough to disregard other therapies that are also effective for various patient populations.

Session Structure

The structure of a BMGIM session is standardized regardless of patient population. Bonny (1978a) lists the four elements of the BMGIM session as preliminary conversation, induction, music listening, and postsession integration or review. The preliminary conversation sets the tone of the sessions and provides an opportunity for the therapist to establish rapport with the client. During this conversation, the therapist assesses the patient's history and major concerns. During the first session, the client is also informed of the BMGIM process and the possible range of imagery experiences.

Following the completion of client history and establishment of treatment goals, the therapist leads the client in an induction that includes two primary elements: relaxation and concentration. Bonny (1975) discovered in the early development of BMGIM that relaxation was necessary for the client to enter the imagination process. Two common types of relaxation are used: a progressive tension-relaxation exercise or an autogenic relaxation. During the preliminary conversation, the therapist must decide which relaxation exercise is appropriate for the client. The relaxation exercise and induction are chosen based on the iso-principle. For example, if a client enters the session in a highly anxious state, the therapist can illustrate the contrast between relaxation and tension by leading the client through a progressive relaxation exercise. Additionally, if the client is psychologically defensive, the therapist can employ an autogenic relaxation exercise to instill in the client a sense of control and comfort.

During progressive relaxation, a person tenses, holds, and then releases large muscle groups. The therapist structures the progression of tension and release to be predictable, and thus encourages relaxation. A possible progression might be relaxation of feet, calves, thighs, pelvis and buttocks, abdomen, chest, back, arms, hands, shoulders, neck, and face. Ideally, the voice of the therapist reflects the stages of tensing, holding, and releasing while providing instructions to the client. The therapist instructions might use the following format: "Tense the muscles in your feet. Tense them and hold them tight. Hold. Hold. Hold. (Pause) Now release. Release completely. Let the tensions go." As the exercise progresses, the client is encouraged to take deep breaths for additional release. After the client has tensed and relaxed all of large muscle groups, he or she tenses the entire body and then releases.

Autogenic relaxation is the use of images to increase client relaxation and concentration. The therapist chooses imagery descriptions based on the client needs or mood states. For example, if a client expresses the need for increased safety and emotional support, the therapist describes an image that illustrates such an experience, such as:

> Imagine that there is a small ball of light resting on the top of your feet. This ball of light can bring to your body a feeling of warmth and relaxation. Let this ball begin to slowly roll from your feet to your calves. As it touches your calves, imagine that it can bring a feeling of warmth and relaxation to them. Let your calves feel that warmth and relaxation from the ball. Now let the ball roll slowly over your knees. [Continue in the same fashion.]

After the relaxation exercise, the therapist provides a bridge to the music listening by describing an opening imagery scene. This bridge or induction creates objects for the client to concentrate on during the music-listening portion of the session. Again, the client issues, mood, and energy level should be considered before the therapist describes the opening imagery scene. With autogenic relaxation, the image used during relaxation can also be the bridge to the music portion of the session. An example might be:

> Now image the small ball of light is cradled in both of your hands. Take a close look at this ball of light; notice the color, texture, form, and anything else that is noticeable. Touch it and feel the sensations. Look into it and notice what is inside. [From this point

the therapist makes a comment that introduces the beginning of the music.] As the music begins, let it explore the light with you, and let it bring you whatever it is you need.

Following the bridge, the music recording is started. The music listening lasts 30 to 40 minutes. During this time, the client listens to the music and orally reports the imagery to the therapist. The therapist is there to support and encourage the client, and to provide the client with the opportunity to explore all of the sensory experiences possible within the imagery. Approaches used to encourage the imagery experience include basic counseling skills such as reflection and empathy. No interpretation of the imagery is given during or after the session, but the therapist must maintain contact with the client through clarification, verbal encouragement, and empathic statements (Bonny, 1978a).

There are three stages during the music-listening portion of the session: the prelude, the bridge, and the heart of the session (Bonny, 1978a). Quickly changing images characterize the prelude. Variations in the imagery may mirror the variations in the music, or sparse imagery may occur with just an occasional symbol or series of thoughts. Possible experiences include, but are not limited to, images from motion pictures or television programs, nature scenes, geometric shapes, matrices of color, or emotions.

The transition from the prelude to the bridge is evident when the client becomes more involved with the imagery process. The transition may be represented by a sense of falling, flying through the air, or walking up or down a stairway. During the transition, imagery can also include crevices, holes, tunnels, caves, or any type of opening. Some clients, especially those who are depressed, report walking in a slow, heavy manner that lasts long enough to facilitate frustration. This frustration is to be encouraged by the therapist, because anger may begin to surface that in turn will motivate the client to change behavior. After the bridge, the heart or goal of the message may become apparent.

After the music listening, the therapist and the client take time to review the imagery experience and to explore how the imagery relates to the client-stated needs and treatment goals. The therapist does not offer an interpretation of the imagery, but encourages the client to draw parallels and meaning from imagery into his or her own life. If the therapist interprets the imagery by projecting issues into the client experience, the client may perceive a lack of empathy from the therapist. In allowing the client to generate his or her own meanings, the client will gain the independence and confidence needed to engage in self-examination.

There can be some variation in the post-session integration depending on the therapist's theoretical orientation. Some therapists may have a client draw to integrate the experience and make it more concrete. Other therapists may verbally integrate the material and do some cognitive work related to the imagery experience. Therapists have also used music improvisation and movement during this portion of the session.

Clinical Applications

The efficacy of BMGIM as a primary therapy modality may be explained by music's nonverbal nature and its ability to elicit memories and feelings. Additionally, music assists clients in lengthening their attention span, sustaining mood, and creating and relieving tension (Jarvis, 1988). Walker (1993) discusses the benefits of integrating verbal psychotherapy and

BMGIM therapy. She states that clients can describe the BMGIM experience to their verbal psychotherapists, so that the material can be included in their therapy. When working with this type of collaborative relationship, it is important that therapists know and agree how to work with the imagery experiences.

The BMGIM process facilitates a very in-depth look at internal struggles; therefore, clients who possess weak egos need additional structure that might not be given to someone who is looking for self-understanding and actualization. Clients involved in BMGIM need to be able to image and discern reality from fantasy. Overtly psychotic persons are not appropriate for this approach. Clients who have thought disorders without formal diagnosis are not difficult to identify; the imagery becomes garish and disconnected. The therapist should refer these clients for further assessment and medication. The therapist needs to be cognizant that this approach may not be the best intervention for all individuals. Some clients may have adverse reactions to the idea of imagery experiences due to religious affiliations and beliefs.

Wrangsjö and Körlin's (1995) study measured changes in psychiatric symptoms. The clients involved in this study exhibited a decrease in most psychiatric symptoms and a significant decrease in interpersonal problems. Clients also identified their lives as more manageable and meaningful. The authors contend that as the client "learns to gather power and nurturance, the client may move deeper into painful and conflictual images and thereby increase his or her competence in handling the inner world, reflected in an increase in manageability" (p. 89). Although the group of subjects in this study was small and heterogeneous, the results seem promising. Even though it did not include a control group, this study seems to suggest that the BMGIM approach may be effective as a primary psychotherapy.

References

Abrams, B. (2002). Transpersonal dimensions of the Bonny Method. In K. E. Bruscia & D. E. Grocke (Eds.), *Guided Imagery and Music: The Bonny Method and beyond*. Gilsum, NH: Barcelona Press.

Association for Music and Imagery (AMI). (2008a). *Core elements of the Bonny Method of Guided Imagery and Music*. Retrieved May 23, 2008, from http://www.ami-bonnymethod.org/docs/core_elements.pdf

Association for Music and Imagery (AMI). (2008b). *Frequently asked questions*. Retrieved May 23, 2008, from http://www.ami-bonnymethod.org/faq.asp

Bonny, H. L. (1972). *Preferred records for use in LSD therapy*. Unpublished report. Maryland Psychiatric Research Center.

Bonny, H. L. (1975). Music and consciousness. *Journal of Music Therapy, 12,* 121–135.

Bonny, H. L. (1978a). *Facilitating Guided Imagery and Music sessions* (GIM Monograph No. 1). Baltimore: ICM Books.

Bonny, H. L. (1978b). *The role of taped music programs in the GIM process* (GIM Monograph No. 2). Baltimore: ICM Books.

Bonny, H. L., & Pahnke, W. N. (1972). The use of music in psychedelic (LSD) psychotherapy. *Journal of Music Therapy, 9,* 62–87.

Bonny, H. L., & Savary L. M. (1990). *Music and your mind: Listening with a new consciousness* (2nd ed.). New York: Statlon Hill Press.

Burns, D. S. (2000). The effects of music on the absorption and control of mental imagery. *Journal of the Association of Mental Imagery, 7,* 39–50.

Goldberg, F. S. (1992). Images of emotion: The role of emotion in Guided Imagery and Music. *Journal of the Association for Music and Imagery, 1,* 5–17.

Goldberg, F. S. (1995). The Bonny Method of Guided Imagery and Music. In T. Wigram, B. Saperston, & R. West (Eds.), *The art and science of music therapy: A handbook* (pp. 112–128). Amsterdam: Overseas Publishers Association.

Goldberg, F. S. (2002). A holographic field theory model of the Bonny Method of Guided Imagery and Music (BMGIM). In K. E. Bruscia & D. E. Grocke (Eds.), *Guided Imagery and Music: The Bonny Method and beyond.* Gilsum, NH: Barcelona Press.

Jarvis, J. (1988). Guided Imagery and Music as a primary psychotherapeutic approach. *Music Therapy Perspectives, 5,* 69–72.

Landau, S. I. (2003). *The new Webster's concise dictionary of the English language* (2003 ed.). Naples, FL: Trident Press International.

Maslow, A. H. (1968). *Toward a psychology of being.* New York: Van Nostrand Reinhold.

McKinney, C. (1990). The effect of music on imagery. *Journal of Music Therapy, 27,* 34–46.

McKinney, C., & Tims, F. (1995). Differential effects of selected classical music on the imagery of high versus low imagers: Two studies. *Journal of Music Therapy, 32,* 22–45.

Peach, S. (1984). Some applications for the clinical use of Guided Imagery and Music. *Journal of Music Therapy, 21,* 27–34.

Quittner, A., & Glueckauf, R. (1983). The facilitative effects of music on visual imagery: A multiple measures approach. *Journal of Mental Imagery, 7,* 105–119.

Rinker, R. L (1991). Guided Imagery and Music (GIM): Healing the wounded healer. In K. E. Bruscia (Ed.), *Case studies in music therapy* (pp. 309–320). Phoenixville, PA: Barcelona.

Ruud, E. (1980). *Music therapy and its relationship to current treatment theories.* St. Louis, MO: MMB Music.

Summer, L. (1993). Melding musical and psychological process: The therapeutic musical space. *Journal of the Association for Music and Imagery, 4,* 37–48.

Vaughan, F. (1979). *Awakening intuition.* New York: Doubleday.

Walker, V. (1993). Integrating Guided Imagery and Music with verbal psychotherapy: A case study. *Journal of the Association for Music and Imagery, 2,* 15–22.

Wrangsjö, B., & Körlin, D. (1995). Guided Imagery and Music as a psychotherapeutic method in psychiatry. *Journal of the Association for Music and Imagery, 4,* 79–92.

Recommended Additional Readings

Bonny, H. L. (1980). *GIM therapy: Past, present, and future implications* (GIM Monograph No. 3). Salina, KS: The Bonny Foundation.

Bonny, H. L. (2002). *Music consciousness: The evolution of Guided Imagery and Music.* Gilsum, NH: Barcelona.

Bonny, H. L., & Bruscia, K. (1996). *Music for the imagination.* Gilsum, NH: Barcelona.

Bruscia, K. E. (1995). The many dimensions of transference. *Journal of the Association for Music and Imagery, 4,* 3–16.

Bruscia, K. E. (1995). Manifestations of transference in Guided Imagery and Music. *Journal of the Association for Music and Imagery, 4,* 17–36.

Bruscia, K. E., & Grocke, D. E. (Eds.). (2002). *Guided Imagery and Music: The Bonny Method and beyond.* Gilsum, NH: Barcelona.

Bush, C. A. (1995). *Healing imagery and music: Pathways to the inner self.* Portland, OR: Rudra Press.

Jacobi, E., & Eisenberg, G. (1994). *The efficacy of the Bonny Method of Guided Imagery and Music (GIM) as experiential therapy in the primary care of persons with rheumatoid arthritis.* Paper presented at the Association for Music and Imagery Conference, Little Switzerland, NC.

Kasayka, R. (1991). *To meet and match the moment of hope: Transpersonal elements of the Guided Imagery and Music experience.* Unpublished doctoral dissertation, New York University.

Logan, H. (1998). *Applied music-evoked imagery for the oncology patient: Results and case studies of a three month music therapy pilot program.* Unpublished manuscript.

McKinney, C., Antoni, M., Kumar, A., & Kumar, M. (1995). Effects of Guided Imagery and Music on depression and beta-endorphin levels in healthy adults: A pilot study. *Journal of the Association for Music and Imagery, 4,* 67–78.

McKinney, C., Antoni, M., Kumar, M., Tims, F., & McCabe, P. (1997). The effects of Guided Imagery and Music (GIM) therapy on mood and cortisol in healthy adults. *Health Psychology, 16,* 390–400.

McKinney, C., Tims, F., Kumar, A., & Kumar, M. (1997). The effect of selected classical music and spontaneous imagery on plasma beta-endorphin. *Journal of Behavioral Medicine, 20,* 85–99.

Stokes, S. J. (1992). Letting the sound depths arise. *Journal of the Association for Music and Imagery, 1,* 69–76.

Summer, L. (1992). Music: The aesthetic elixir. *Journal of the Association for Music and Imagery, 1,* 43–54.

Toomey, L. (1996–1997). Literature review: The Bonny Method of Guided Imagery and Music. *Journal of the Association for Music and Imagery, 5,* 75–103.

Wrangsjö, B. (1995). Psychoanalysis and Guided Imagery and Music: A comparison. *Journal of the Association for Music and Imagery, 4,* 35–48.

Chapter 6

Nordoff-Robbins Music Therapy

Kenneth Aigen
Cari Kennedy Miller
Youngshin Kim
Varvara Pasiali
Eum-Mi Kwak
Daniel B. Tague

Overview

Nordoff-Robbins Music Therapy originated from the teamwork of Paul Nordoff and Clive Robbins. Paul Nordoff, an American composer and pianist, and Clive Robbins, a British-trained special educator, collaborated for 17 years, from 1959 until Nordoff's death in 1976. Robbins also collaborated with his wife, Carol Matteson Robbins, from 1975 until her death in 1996. Nordoff-Robbins Music Therapy is an active, creative, improvisational approach to therapy. It is based on the belief that within every human being resides an inborn musicality that can be activated in the service of personal growth and development.

This self-actualizing potential is most effectively awakened through the use of improvisational music in which the individual's innate creativity is used to overcome emotional, physical, and cognitive difficulties. In this form of co-creative endeavor, clients take an active role in creating music together with their therapists on a variety of standard and specialized instruments. Because instruments that are expressively gratifying yet do not require special skills to play can be chosen, no prior experience or training in music is required of clients.

There are Nordoff-Robbins Music Therapy organizations and centers in Australia, England, Germany, New York, New Zealand, and Scotland. Organizations devoted to its study and dissemination exist in Japan and Korea. The Nordoff-Robbins communities in each of these countries continue to develop clinical work, research, instructional publications, and musical repertoire. This chapter begins with a discussion of the historical background of Nordoff-Robbins therapy and its philosophical and theoretical orientations. It continues with an explanation of the Nordoff-Robbins clinical training and ends with a detailed description of Nordoff-Robbins Music Therapy and its clinical uses.

History

Paul Nordoff was a graduate of the Philadelphia Conservatory of Music and the Julliard Graduate School of Music. He was professor of composition and piano at Bard College from 1949 to 1958 and received several awards for his compositions. During a sabbatical in 1958 in Europe, Nordoff witnessed the ability of children with disabilities to respond to music, and he recognized that music had a therapeutic power. In 1959, Nordoff gave up his academic career as a musician and joined in researching the power of music for the handicapped at Sunfield Children's Home in England (Nordoff-Robbins Center for Music Therapy, 2001c). Sunfield Children's Home is a residential school for emotionally and intellectually disabled children and adolescents. The theoretical side of Sunfield Children's Home program was based on anthroposophical principles, and the practical side of the program focused on art therapies as practiced by various specialists: music, eurhythmy, painting, modeling, musical theater, puppet theater, and handcrafts. In 1959 and 1960 at Sunfield, Nordoff began his work with the assistance of Clive Robbins, who was working as a special class teacher. They made a natural team for they had much in common, such as anthroposophical backgrounds and a profound respect for each child with whom they worked (Hadley, 1998). At this stage, Nordoff and Robbins experimentally developed their work for the practical purpose. They studied and analyzed how musical elements such as intervals, consonance-dissonance, rhythms, vibrato, and scale tonality affected the children's responses, and they began developing the foundations of Nordoff-Robbins Music Therapy (Nordoff & Robbins, 1992).

From June to November 1960, Nordoff and Robbins visited 24 institutions for children with special needs in England, Scotland, Sweden, Denmark, Holland, Germany, and Switzerland to gain comparative experiences of music offerings at different educational and residential settings. However, this tour turned into a lecture-demonstration tour as they worked with a wide variety of children at each home they visited (Aigen, 1998). Following the tour, Nordoff and Robbins began their work in the United States in 1961 with pilot projects at the Daycare Unit for Autistic Children, Department of Child Psychiatry, School of Medicine, University of Pennsylvania, and the Devereux Foundation. At the Daycare Unit, they worked with children who presented autism, developmental disabilities, multiple disabilities, or emotional disturbances. They developed their approach further while working with children with physical and communication disabilities at the Institute of Logopedics in Wichita, Kansas (Nordoff-Robbins Center for Music Therapy, 2001c). Their first book, *Therapy in Music for Handicapped Children*, published by Rudolf Steiner Publications in 1965, describes Nordoff and Robbins's work at Sunfield Children's Home in England and observations from their European tour in 1960 and outlines the musical explorations at the Daycare Unit for Autistic Children and the Institute of Logopedics. This book was expanded in 1971, the title was changed to *Therapy in Music for Handicapped Children*, and it is currently available under this title (Nordoff & Robbins, 2004).

The effectiveness of music therapy impressed the multidisciplinary team directing the program at the Daycare Unit for Autistic Children. The members of the multidisciplinary team applied to the National Institute of Mental Health (NIMH) to acquire funding for their work. As a result, NIMH approved a comprehensive 3-year project including treatment, research, training, and publication. In 1965, NIMH granted supplementary funding for an additional 2 years (the Daycare Unit was now called the Developmental Center for Autistic Children, Inc., Philadelphia). The 5-year music therapy project (May 1962 to May 1967) was called "Music

Therapy Project for Psychotic Children Under Seven." The book *Creative Music Therapy* described the responses of children who participated in the project and provided a comprehensive view of the creative music therapy process (Nordoff & Robbins, 1977).

Two associate superintendents of the School District of Philadelphia observed music therapy sessions at the Daycare Unit of the University of Pennsylvania in June 1962. They acknowledged the potential of music therapy in special education. Because of their support, Nordoff and Robbins conducted a music therapy project with the Board of Public Education of the School District of Philadelphia from 1962 to 1967. In 1967, they began a series of workshops and seminars in all five Scandinavian countries, sponsored by the American-Scandinavian Foundation and the Finnish National Welfare Association for the Mentally Deficient. For the next 7 years, Nordoff and Robbins combined international traveling, teaching, and lecturing with writing their three major books: *Creative Music Therapy* (1977), *Music Therapy in Special Education* (1983)*,* and *Therapy in Music for Handicapped Children* (1992)*. Music Therapy in Special Education* was based on a series of manuals compiled for special education teachers in the public schools of Philadelphia and resource materials prepared for participants in music therapy workshops and seminars given in the Scandinavian countries (Nordoff & Robbins, 1983).

In 1975, Clive Robbins began work with his wife, Carol Robbins, at the New York State School for the Deaf at Rome. Carol Robbins was an accomplished musician and teacher who had begun studying with Nordoff and Robbins in 1966. Clive Robbins and his wife adapted the Nordoff-Robbins Music Therapy approach for children with hearing impairments and demonstrated the effectiveness of music in stimulating the use of residual hearing. Their "Music Curriculum for the Deaf" project was federally funded for 3 years (Nordoff-Robbins Center for Music Therapy, 2001c). During that time, through a series of treatment and clinical research projects, the Robbins-Robbins team developed musical techniques and resources for both individual and group therapy for children with hearing impairments. Their book *Music for the Hearing Impaired and Other Special Groups: A Resource Manual and Curriculum Guide,* published in 1980, describes the findings of the project.

In 1975, the Nordoff-Robbins Music Therapy Centre was established in London as the first facility devoted to Nordoff-Robbins Music Therapy. Therapists at the London Centre began applying the Nordoff-Robbins approach in new treatment contexts, such as in adult psychiatric and geriatric settings. In Germany, Nordoff-Robbins therapists began working in 1978 at the Community Hospital, Herdecke. This development eventually resulted in the establishment of The Institute for Music Therapy at the University of Witten/Herdecke in 1985. The institute staff extended the Nordoff-Robbins approach into new areas such as pediatrics, spinal cord injuries, neurology, and intensive care.

Clive and Carol Robbins founded the Nordoff-Robbins Center for Music Therapy at New York University in 1989. The center provides music therapy services for clients, and training and seminars for music therapists and students; prepares instructional materials; and undertakes and publishes qualitative research. Carol Robbins codirected the center with her husband until her passing in 1996. In 1998, Clive Robbins moved to the position of founding director, and Kenneth Aigen and Alan Turry became codirectors of the center. Aigen left the center in 2006, and Turry remains as the Executive Director. Clive Robbins remains active as a teacher and lecturer on an international basis.

Currently, organizations offering Nordoff-Robbins Music Therapy services exist in England, Scotland, Germany, Australia, New Zealand, and New York. An organization devoted to its study—the Organization for the Study of Nordoff-Robbins Music Therapy (OSNRMT)—exists in Japan. In addition, there are trained Nordoff-Robbins therapists working in several other countries, including Korea and Greece. There is also an International Trust for Nordoff-Robbins Music Therapy, incorporated in the U.K. but consisting of members from a number of countries. This organization regulates the international use of the "Nordoff-Robbins" name in clinical and training programs and controls the use of the original Nordoff-Robbins clinical archives and publications.

In recent years, there have been a number of publications detailing different aspects of the history of Nordoff-Robbins Music Therapy and of the primary individuals involved in its development and dissemination. Interested readers are directed to the appreciation of the life of Carol Robbins by Clive Robbins (Robbins, 1997), the research study by Susan Hadley (1998), the autobiography of Clive Robbins (Robbins, 2005), and the historical text by Fraser Simpson (2007) that focuses on the story of Nordoff-Robbins Music Therapy with an emphasis on its evolution in the United Kingdom.

Philosophical and Theoretical Orientations

The theoretical foundations of Nordoff-Robbins music therapy are congruent with a variety of ideas in psychology and the philosophy of music. Paul Nordoff invoked the philosophy of music advocated by Victor Zuckerkandl in his early music therapy teachings (Aigen, 1996). Supportive ideas on the nature of music and its role in human development were based on principles of anthroposophy according to Rudolf Steiner. Abraham Maslow's (1968) concept of self-actualization provided an appropriate concept to summarize views of human development that Nordoff and Robbins had arrived at independently from their experiences of the extraordinary clinical efficacy of creative music therapy (Bruscia, 1987). Although their work did not originate in Steiner's teaching directly, certain areas of anthroposophical thinking and values supported the origination of their approach. The worldview in anthroposophy had influenced their attitude of reverence for the meaningfulness of human destiny. Based on this shared belief, Nordoff and Robbins respected the inner life of each child with whom they worked and had an open vision toward exploring the powers of music to reach the unknown developmental potentials latent in disabled children (Robbins, 1993).

Moreover, like Steiner, Nordoff and Robbins believed that within every human being is a musical self that responds to music, resonates with emotions, and mirrors other aspects of the personality, which they referred to as the "music child" (Nordoff & Robbins, 2007). Nordoff and Robbins stated:

> The *music child* is therefore the individualized musicality inborn in every child: the term has reference to the universality of human musical sensitivity—the heritage of complex and subtle sensitivity to the ordering and relationship of tonal and rhythmic movement—and to the uniquely personal significance of each child's musical responsiveness. (p. 1)

Nordoff and Robbins believed that an active music-making process could awaken the "music child" in a child with special needs, which is blocked because of one's handicapped condition.

The awakening of the "music child" increases the individual's self-awareness and allows an individual to discover meaning and joy in the therapeutic experience, which leads to developing communicative intention in his or her musical response (Nordoff & Robbins, 1977).

Just as Steiner believed the soul of man should be reviewed and then described in musical terms, Nordoff and Robbins believed that musical experiences should mirror one's psychological and developmental conditions (Bruscia, 1987). They believed that the ability of an individual to experience emotional awareness, form and order, tempo, rhythm, and song increased as the receptive, cognitive, and expressive capabilities of the "music child" within the individual's own personality became more organized (Nordoff & Robbins, 1977). Thus, "ideally after participating in this musical relationship, the client is able to participate in his or her environment in a fuller, more complete way" (Turry, 1998).

Prior to the development of the theoretical concept of the "music child," the ideas of anthroposophy influenced the practical use of music in Nordoff-Robbins Music Therapy. Nordoff and Robbins valued Steiner's concept of music intervals and musical archetypes and used them in clinical improvisation. Steiner believed each interval evokes its own creative experience. For example, a minor second creates "an inward experience, but with a stirring of movement and activity within the self" (Bruscia, 1987, p. 31). In addition, Nordoff-Robbins therapists use the complete range of musical styles and scales that exist internationally from a belief that different styles and scales have inherent qualities that can resonate with the client's inner life and provide an external portrait of the client's inner self (Turry, 1998). References to the musical influences of anthroposophy can be found in several Nordoff-Robbins texts: in *Healing Heritage,* Explorations Four to Six—musical intervals; and in Exploration Fourteen— the archetypal nature of musical idioms and styles (Robbins & Robbins, 1998). Such influences are also found in Aigen's (1998) research study of eight seminal clients seen by the original Nordoff-Robbins team—*Paths of Development in Nordoff-Robbins Music Therapy.* These influences are particularly evident in the study "Goodbye Indu" in the context of the use of mirror-image scales, and in the study "Audrey is Dancing a Song"—the use of a fairy tale in therapy (Aigen, 1998).

The publications of Nordoff and Robbins focused on the "music child," and those of Robbins and Robbins expanded this conceptual focus to include some of Abraham H. Maslow's humanistic concepts. Clive Robbins connected Maslow's humanistic psychology with his work in 1973, which was made public in 1976 (Robbins, 1993). The connection emerged when Clive Robbins was searching for a psychologically acceptable theory that fit into the psychological foundation of Nordoff-Robbins Music Therapy. Maslow believed in developing a person's strengths and potentials rather than focusing on one's deficiencies. Robbins and Robbins thought that this idea best described the growth-motivated approach of Nordoff-Robbins Music Therapy, which leads to self-actualization and peak experiences (Bruscia, 1987). They also believed in intrinsic learning, which creates opportunities for individuals to take emotional risks, make choices with ease, engage in self-expression, and discover their strengths and weaknesses. Last, Robbins and Robbins valued Maslow's concept of one's self-actualizing creativeness, which stems from the personal qualities of "courage, boldness, freedom, spontaneity, integration, and self-acceptance" (Bruscia, 1987, p. 33).

Even though the Nordoff-Robbins Music Therapy approach was originally developed with children with disabilities, when the work developed beyond the original team, it expanded to include adults as well, including those under medical, psychiatric, and geriatric care. In addition, some Nordoff-Robbins therapists also work with adults who seek to overcome emotional difficulties or achieve personal growth. Working with individuals without severe disabilities has motivated therapists to integrate psychotherapy constructs, theories, and practices into their overall approach. As a result, there is a wide spectrum of beliefs among clinicians and theorists of Nordoff-Robbins Music Therapy. Some clinicians feel comfortable using psychotherapy practices such as making interpretations, gaining insight, and examining the dynamics of the therapist-client relationship. Other clinicians believe that the music-centered characteristics of the Nordoff-Robbins approach make transfers from verbally based forms of therapy unnecessary or even inappropriate. "They believe that describing the processes comprising creative clinical improvisation through psychological constructs necessarily distorts the essence of the musical interaction" (Turry, 1998). To integrate the two extremes, some theorists have attempted to interpret the musical improvisations that occur during a session as manifestations of traditional psychotherapeutic phenomena. Several issues regarding the relationship between Nordoff-Robbins' work and the practices of verbal psychotherapy are currently receiving scholarly discussion (Nordoff-Robbins Center for Music Therapy, 2001b); these can be found in the Newsletter of the International Association of Nordoff-Robbins Therapists called *Musicing,* as well as in a series of articles from the *British Journal of Music Therapy* by Aigen (1999), Ansdell (1999), Brown (1999), Pavlicevic (1999), and Streeter (1999).

Training

The Nordoff-Robbins Center at New York University is the only facility in the United States where therapists can learn the Nordoff-Robbins approach. The center offers an internship program for students enrolled in graduate study in music therapy. The internship program is 38 weeks long, requires a minimum of 25 hours of clinical and course work per week, and includes (a) classes in clinical musicianship, improvisation, and the practice and theory of group music therapy; (b) clinical work and documentation in individual and group therapy; and (c) weekly individual clinical supervision. The certification program, called Level One Training, leads to the designation NRMT (Nordoff-Robbins Music Therapist) and is open for professional music therapists who already have a master's degree in music therapy or credentialed music therapists who are concurrently enrolled in a master's program. It is not necessary to complete an academic internship at the NR Center in order to apply for the Certification Training Program. The length of training for Level One certification ranges from 1 to 2 years. Acceptance requirements include prior clinical experience and use of improvisation in clinical work. All applicants for the training course must audition and interview with the training personnel. Certification candidates take the same classes as the internship program students. In addition, they participate in advanced seminars and workshops and may take supplemental classes within the New York University master's program (Nordoff-Robbins Center for Music Therapy, 2001a, 2001e).

Level Two Training consists of ongoing clinical supervision, case presentations to colleagues and professional audiences, instructional seminars, and exchanges with other Nordoff-Robbins therapists in the United States and abroad. Level Three Training is open to therapists who have completed the previous two levels of training. Completion of Level Three Training qualifies individuals to be a Head of Training at a Nordoff-Robbins facility (Nordoff-Robbins Center for Music Therapy, 2001e).

Description of Nordoff-Robbins Music Therapy

Clinical Setting

The Nordoff-Robbins therapeutic setting often depends on available resources and needs of the client. Initially, the Nordoff-Robbins approach utilized two therapists working as a team. The primary therapist improvises at the piano or the guitar to engage the child in a therapeutic music experience, while the co-therapist works directly with the client to facilitate responses. When working as part of a team, the primary therapist continues to be responsible for the music and the overall direction of therapy. The co-therapist facilitates the musical interaction and supports the primary therapist's clinical focus and the client's efforts. However, having two therapists for each session is not always practical or clinically appropriate. In some cases, more than two therapists work together for a larger group or with a group whose members have severe physical challenges and need physical assistance. In other cases, a therapist works alone, such as is the case with children who do not require the support of a co-therapist or nonpathological adults (Turry, 1998).

Based on individual needs, the client may participate in individual therapy, group therapy, or both. Individual therapy may be appropriate for clients who are minimally responsive to the therapy situation, are noncommunicative, or have behaviors that interfere with peer interaction or participation in a group musical activity. On the other hand, some clients exhibit special musical skills and sensitivities and are recommended to individual therapy in order to get the full benefits that such individualized attention can provide. Thus, while some clients do develop skills in individual therapy that prepare them for subsequent group work, the developmental process of therapy does not inevitably have to move from individual to group work.

If the client needs peer support and modeling in order to further responses, group therapy is appropriate. Group therapy may be supplemental to individual therapy, allowing the client to enhance and apply communication skills and personal autonomy attained in the individual setting. When the client begins to demonstrate communicative behaviors, which are necessary for the group setting, the client may be making significant therapeutic growth. If the client in individual therapy appears to reach a plateau and needs increased social stimulation, he or she may benefit from group therapy (Bruscia, 1987). And for many clients, creating music in a group setting provides experiences of community that they may not be able to acquire in any other way. Giving this experience of belonging to something larger than oneself is an essential part of all music therapy group placements.

Clinical Environment

The environment for therapy sessions should be acoustically welcoming and equipped with quality musical instruments. Typically, the therapist's primary instrument is the piano or the guitar, because such harmonic instruments allow for the musical flexibility and the creation of a variety of musical styles and moods essential to the efficacy of Nordoff-Robbins work.

Traditionally, the piano has been widely used for primary therapists. However, during the 1990s, some contemporary Nordoff-Robbins practitioners began using the guitar, as it was their primary instrument. In addition, the therapist's use of the voice is absolutely essential, both in singing words and as an instrument in its own right. Often, the voice as an instrument is used in a way to musically complement what the therapist is playing on the guitar or piano. Because they are used with a variety of fixed pitch instruments, the piano or guitar should be accurately tuned and have a good quality of sound.

Clients use any and all instruments, with a focus on those that are of high quality, do not require specialized training to play, and offer a variety of expressive possibilities. Practically, this often involves the use of all types of wooden and metal pitched percussion instruments; all kinds of drums, cymbals, and gongs; the piano; and string instruments such as harps, cellos, and guitars, some of which are specially adapted, such as using a single string cello or guitars that are tuned to open chords. In addition, some clients express themselves primarily with the voice through lyrics and nonverbal singing. Movement and dancing are seen as expressive acts as well and are incorporated into the therapist's music. Electric guitars and keyboards are used also, as are full drum sets, especially when the client's musical expression or preference tends toward contemporary popular idioms such as rock or jazz.

Treatment Process

Due to its music-centered philosophy, in the Nordoff-Robbins approach music serves as the primary clinical medium and agent of change. This does not imply that therapists do not speak with their clients or do not do important therapeutic work verbally when this is in the client's best interest. It does mean that there is a belief that musical interaction and expression provide unique clinical benefits that cannot be achieved through verbal means, and thus therapists are always conscious of guiding their clients into music and helping them to work on clinical issues through the music.

In improvising and playing precomposed pieces, therapists use the elements of music with conscious clinical intent. Things such as the direction and overall construction of melodies, the degree and type of dissonance, the use of cadences, the use of specific styles and scales, and even the therapist's touch and timbre are all chosen very directly to enhance the therapist's ability to musically connect with the client, engage the client in the music, and then provide challenging opportunities for client growth through co-improvised music (Turry, 1998). Although music is primarily improvised in most sessions, prewritten pieces are often used. Compositions designed specifically for use in therapy can be found in songbooks such as *Play Songs* 1 through 5, *Themes for Therapy, More Themes for Therapy, Greetings and Goodbyes,* and similar collections. Complete reference information for these resources can be found in the list of Musical Resources located at the end of this chapter.

There is no prescribed format or series of procedures when therapist and client work together musically. As the therapist responds and creates music with the client, he or she is also assessing the client's needs. For one client, sparse nonpulsed music may be utilized to create an inviting space for the client to enter into. For another client, pulse-driven stimulating music that contains dissonances may be utilized immediately. The therapist works to bring challenges that guide clients to their developmental threshold, utilizing elements of music that both support and challenge. The client responds to the therapist and the therapist responds to the client's response, thus building a musical form and direction between them. The therapist creates music that enhances the client's musical expression, hoping to support a wider and more varied expression on the part of the client.

Establishing musical communication between the client and the therapist can be an important goal. The therapist improvises music that matches, accompanies, and enhances the client's emotions from moment to moment. By matching the client's mood, the therapist is not only creating an accepting and trusting atmosphere, but also enhancing the potential for musical direction and interaction. Unpredictable and unfamiliar music is often used to stimulate interest and intrigue the client in order to increase his or her engagement. At times the music can be quite intrusive. The process is one of trial and error that is balanced with careful indexing of the client responses, which takes place after each session. For clients who have difficulty communicating, evoking musical responses from them, vocal or instrumental, can be an important goal. The therapist accepts unconditionally what the client presents as potential musical communication. Often the client develops musical skills by exploring various rhythmic patterns, dynamic changes, melodic and harmonic blends, and tempo changes within the musical improvisations. As a result, the client expands his or her expressive skills. Expanding a client's expressive capability builds self-confidence and increases awareness of "inter-responsiveness," which is the discovery and awareness of the relationship between the music the client makes and the therapist (Bruscia, 1987).

Improvisational Techniques

Since music serves as a primary medium and agent of change in therapy, clinical techniques focus on issues of what kind of music the therapist should play and how it should be played, in order to match, accompany, and enhance a client's response. Most important, the therapist should improvise with clinical intention in a way that makes deliberate use of the aesthetic properties of musical experience. The aesthetic properties, such as the beauty of a melody or the warmth of harmonic accompaniment, are seen as essential to the clinical process for two reasons.

First, all people, regardless of disability, can perceive these qualities, and music of higher aesthetic quality is generally more effective in engaging clients and providing a richer experience to them. Essential to Nordoff-Robbins work is the idea that by connecting to one's inner creative drive, clients can overcome the limitations imposed by disability and trauma. Music of an aesthetic nature is more effective in connecting clients to their own creative capacities.

Second, the music created in Nordoff-Robbins work is seen as an outer manifestation of a client's inner life. The reason why otherwise unresponsive clients respond so well in this approach is because they cannot help but identify with, and feel themselves reflected in, the therapist's music. Therapists endeavor to find the beauty that is the essence of each person and to put this into musical form. Thus, the aesthetic quality of the therapist's music is a direct reflection of both the client's inner being and the way this becomes manifest in the therapeutic relationship through the therapist's individual musical sensitivity. This music is created in mutual fashion as the therapist is basing what he plays on the client's presentation and responses, regardless of whether or not the client is active musically.

And last, saying that the aesthetic properties of music are essential to clinical efficacy does not imply that Nordoff-Robbins therapists exclusively use music that is conventionally "pretty." Much music of a high degree of aesthetic quality can be quite dissonant, harsh, or otherwise challenging. The therapist uses all possible elements of music in all possible combinations to best reflect an individual client's experience of life, something that can demand quite challenging music.

The therapist's music should serve as "clinical" improvisation, which means that it avoids expressing one's own musical preference, feelings, and habitual patterns, but rather it is personalized to the client's emotional state, functions, and needs. Because they have multiple levels of meaning and experience, the clinical interventions through music can be simultaneously challenging and supporting, inviting and demanding, leading and following; they can simultaneously offer all of these things and thus support contact with the child's present functioning level while still providing an invitation to growth (Aigen, 1996).

Moreover, the therapist's music should not be subject to conventional restraints, such as music based on a diatonic scale or typical chord progressions, in order to provide unique individualized musical experience. Thus, the therapist should be familiar with different modes and idioms from various parts of the world and should realize the potential emotional effects of each musical archetype. In addition, the therapist should have the ability to be flexible, to change his or her music in any musical elements, such as tempo, dynamic, meter, key, register, accent, and melodic and harmonic direction, responding to change in a client's music and movement. The improvisation must be progressive so that the therapist continues to develop the improvisational themes from session to session (Nordoff & Robbins, 2007). However, the therapist might need to create new musical material or play the material in a new way if the clinical situation requires change. Improvisations may be created intuitively to meet a client's needs at the moment or material from preexisting compositions or precomposed songs can be incorporated.

Nordoff and Robbins described specific improvisational techniques used during a music therapy session in each of their published books. Bruscia (1987) summarized the techniques that Nordoff-Robbins clinicians implement to match a client's mood. The therapist describes a client's personality using musical improvisations, creates improvisations that suit the mood of the moment, and musically describes the client's facial expression and physical bearing. Additionally, the therapist observes a client's movements and sets them to music; chants songs that describe the client's actions, mood, or experience; and imitates the sounds that the client makes using instruments or voice. Nordoff and Robbins (2007) described several techniques used to evoke vocalizations or singing responses. These techniques include humming, whistling, or singing nonverbal syllables, and chanting word phrases. Techniques used to elicit instrumental responses include imitating the rhythmic patterns that a client presents, introducing tempo changes, isolating melodic and rhythmic motifs out of what the client improvises, presenting short melodic motifs or phrases that end with a rest or on an unresolved tone, or playing a harmonic progression that has not resolved to the tonic, thus inviting completion by the client (Nordoff & Robbins, 2007). In order to evoke response, unresolved or incomplete melodic and harmonic phrases can be created.

Goals and Objectives

Clinical goals and objectives in Nordoff-Robbins Music Therapy aim to develop the client's individual potential rather than the conforming to specific behaviors to meet cultural expectations or universal standards for normality (Nordoff & Robbins, 1992). Instead of forming short-term behavioral objectives, Nordoff-Robbins clinicians focus on long-term therapeutic growth, which is characterized by expressive freedom and creativity, communicativeness, self-confidence, and independence. Their interest in a child's inner life and growth as clinical goals is closely linked to Maslow's theories of creativeness, intrinsic learning, peak experiences, growth motivation, and self-actualization. The changes seen in treatment do not relate merely to a client's outer behavior but to the inner life of perception, thought, and feeling (Nordoff-Robbins Center for Music Therapy, 2001a).

Since music serves primary functions in therapy, clinical goals are attained within musical goals. Nordoff and Robbins (2007) believed that musical growth is therapeutic growth. "Thus, personal freedom is realized through musical freedom; interpersonal communicativeness is realized through musical "inter-responsiveness"; and self-confidence is realized through independent creativity in music" (Bruscia, 1987, p. 27).

Assessment and Data Collection

Nordoff and Robbins believed that assessment and data collection in Nordoff-Robbins Music Therapy provide a musical map of the client and, in turn, direct the course of therapy (Nordoff & Robbins, 1992). The client's musical responses have diagnostic, etiological, or theoretical significance, although psychological interpretations have been "avoided and supplanted by purely descriptive statements of the client's musical communicativeness" (Bruscia, 1987, p. 35). Nordoff-Robbins music therapists usually do not collect data focusing on specific target behaviors. Instead, each session is audio- or video-recorded, then reviewed by the team members (primary therapist and co-therapist) after the session. They study clients' significant musical/nonmusical responses, changes, musical relationship, and teamwork. In a process known as "indexing," sessions are documented in a narrative style in detail with a time basis. Through indexing, therapists are able to focus on moment-to-moment changes in the client and in the music. Often, music created in a session is transcribed during the process, for repetition and possible development in succeeding sessions. Indexing allows therapists to take a more objective view of what happened, assess interventions, and analyze perceptions of the situation from a distance (Turry, 1998). By indexing, therapists gain another perspective on the events of the session.

Reviewing the session recordings provides an objective distance from these events that has both advantages and drawbacks. The advantage is that the therapist can re-experience the client's expression when he or she is not simultaneously concerned with providing an ongoing musical experience for the client; the disadvantage is that in this distancing what is lost is the feeling of being with the client in the music, and this subjective experience of the music is an important aspect of the entire process. Ideally, the therapists endeavor to combine their immediate subjective impressions of the session with the more objective impressions to formulate a more complete sense of the client's clinical process. In a sense, indexing is a form of peer supervision, as therapists help each other to become aware of impediments to the therapy process and to develop new understandings of the clients and their reaction to them.

Besides the commitment to self-monitoring reflected in the process of documentation after each session, Nordoff-Robbins practitioners use several assessment instruments developed by Paul Nordoff and Clive Robbins: *Thirteen Categories of Response, Evaluation Scales I and II, Musical Responses Scale III,* and the *Tempo-Dynamic Schema,* all of which can be found in Nordoff and Robbins (2007). Each assessment instrument provides information pertaining to the musical responses and reactions of clients and allows the therapist to evaluate the client's responses and personal reactions to the improvisational experiences. Nordoff-Robbins clinicians usually do not use all four scales for the same client or for every session. Rather, a particular scale can be carefully chosen based on the area that needs to be evaluated and can be conducted intermittently during the entire course of therapy. The outcomes can be reflected in the modified long-term goals.

Nordoff-Robbins therapists may use the first scale, *Thirteen Categories of Response* (Nordoff & Robbins, 1992), to document each client's musical responses. *Evaluation Scales I and II* measure the client-therapist relationship within the musical activity, as well as the "Musical Communicativeness" that occurs. According to the evaluation scales, the client experiences high levels of therapeutic growth if he or she demonstrates expressive freedom and creativity, communication, self-confidence, and independence. The third scale, *Musical Responses Scale III*, measures musical complexity, expressiveness, and the inter-responsiveness of instrumental and vocal music. Last, the *Tempo-Dynamic Schema* focuses on these elements in the therapists' improvisation, analyzes them, and categorizes their effects in the client-therapists co-activity.

Therapeutic Uses

Nordoff-Robbins therapists work with a broad range of people, including children with disabilities, individuals under psychiatric care, self-referred adults, individuals in medical settings, or older adults in residential home care (Nordoff-Robbins Center for Music Therapy, 2001d). Researchers have used primarily qualitative research methods to investigate the effectiveness of Nordoff-Robbins Music Therapy. In the books they have published, Nordoff and Robbins have included several case studies describing the therapeutic use of Nordoff-Robbins Music Therapy with children who have special needs. Aigen (1995) presented clinical examples using the Nordoff-Robbins approach with two children who had autism and severe developmental disabilities. He has proposed a therapeutic model integrating developmental therapy and music psychotherapy interventions. In another study, Aigen (1998) examined the early work of the original Nordoff-Robbins team and discussed it in light of contemporary issues in music therapy. Moreover, Aldridge, Gustorff, and Neugebauer (1995) have documented the developmental changes displayed by five children with developmental delays who received 3 months of improvisational music therapy, in comparison with three children with developmental delays who served as waiting-list controls.

Various researchers have described the use of Nordoff-Robbins Music Therapy with adolescents. Exploring the intense connection to music of a 17-year-old boy who had developmental delays and a history of sexual abuse, Ritholz and Turry (1994) engaged him into the therapeutic process and increased his creative interactions with others. Aigen (1997) described in detail the group process over the course of 1 year with a group of four adolescents with developmental delays, autism, or both. He explained the various functions of music, including facilitating transitions between activities or at the beginning and closing of the session, meeting group and individual needs of clients, transforming ritualistic motor behaviors into communicative gestures, increasing emotional self-awareness, and enhancing interpersonal relationships.

Current research has indicated that Nordoff-Robbins Music Therapy is effective with adults. In two case studies with adults who had dementia, Ishizuka (1998) explored how Nordoff-Robbins Music Therapy facilitated verbal and nonverbal interaction. By transcribing and analyzing extracts from her work with these clients, the author suggested that even though the clients' speech did not have concrete meaning, the use of improvised music enabled therapists to respond to clients and share emotions and feelings. Moreover, Robel (1997) has described the role of Nordoff-Robbins Music Therapy in increasing motivation of adults in neurological rehabilitation.

Conclusion: Contemporary Developments in Nordoff-Robbins Music Therapy

The Nordoff-Robbins approach is defined more by an attitude to music, creativity, and human potential than by allegiance to a particular approach or nonmusical theoretical belief system. For this reason, it has proved to be unusually malleable in adapting to various cultures, styles of music, and theoretical frameworks. Currently, there is significant activity in countries such as Korea and Japan, and it is expected that Nordoff-Robbins clinical and training programs will eventually be established in these countries. To facilitate this development, several Nordoff-Robbins texts, such as Aigen (1998), Robbins and Robbins (1998), and Ansdell (1995) have been translated into Japanese and Korean.

The seminal text *Creative Music Therapy* has recently been completely revised and expanded in a second edition (Nordoff & Robbins, 2007). The new edition contains twice the amount of text as the original and the amount of audio material has expanded from that which could be provided on a single audio tape to four CDs worth of case examples. While true to the original work, the current version also represents the evolution in Clive Robbins' thinking that occurred during the 30 years between the two publication dates.

Each culture to which Nordoff-Robbins work has been introduced has provided fertile ground for novel applications. In Germany, the work in medical settings continues to develop in innovative ways. Some of these important developments in the medical area can be found in Aldridge (1996), and new ways to use improvisation as a diagnostic tool in dementia can be found in Aldridge (2000). Important music-based research into the nature of melody can be found in Aldridge and Aldridge (2008). Ansdell (1995) also provides an overview of Nordoff-Robbins work with adult clients in various settings and discusses many of the concepts underlying this approach to creative music therapy. Lee (1996) provides a detailed examination of a course of therapy with a musician with HIV/AIDS. Both the Ansdell and Lee publications contain companion audio recordings that are invaluable in helping to communicate the nature of their work. And last, Turry (2007) provides a pioneering research effort that examines the relationship between music and lyric content in the improvised expressions of an adult woman client with cancer.

The approach is also implemented within an increasing diversity of musical styles and theoretical frameworks. In this vein, Lee (2003) advances his notion of Aesthetic Music Therapy, which is an outgrowth of Nordoff-Robbins work that is based upon a variety of traditional and modern compositional resources including atonal music. Aigen (2002/2005) provides a detailed study of improvisational Nordoff-Robbins work using popular idioms such as rock and jazz music, while supplementing traditional Nordoff-Robbins theory with concepts drawn from ethnomusicology. Both works continue the Nordoff-Robbins tradition of making full use of available technology in disseminating knowledge of music therapy, as Lee's book contains a pristine digital audio recording, and Aigen's publication comes with a DVD. Both studies illustrate how Nordoff-Robbins principles are applicable within any musical tradition.

Nordoff-Robbins practice and practitioners continue to influence other streams of development in music therapy, even as they are influenced by these avenues of thought. Pavlicevic (1997) examines a number of crucial issues in music therapy through the lenses of three particular focuses: music theory and music psychology, theories on the relation of music and emotion, and psychodynamic theory. Ansdell (2002) and Pavlicevic and Ansdell (2004) both discuss the notion of "Community Music Therapy" as a contemporary movement that establishes a framework for music therapy practice that goes beyond traditional boundaries in terms of interventions, milieu, and clients. Aigen (2005) establishes a theoretical foundation for music-centered music therapy, thus taking the principles that have supported the Nordoff-Robbins work and putting them in a more general form to be applied within other forms of practice. In closing, these contemporary developments illustrate one of the prime values of a music-centered music therapy approach. Such a pragmatic commitment to the value of musical interaction and expression ensures the continued relevance of the Nordoff-Robbins approach in a world characterized by constant change.

References

Aigen, K. (1995). Cognitive and affective processes in music therapy with individuals with developmental delays: A preliminary model for contemporary Nordoff-Robbins practice. *Music Therapy, 13,* 13–45.

Aigen, K. (1996). *Being in music: Foundations of Nordoff-Robbins Music Therapy.* The Nordoff-Robbins Music Therapy Monograph Series (Vol. 1). Gilsum, NH: Barcelona.

Aigen, K. (1997). *Here we are in music: One year with an adolescent creative music therapy group.* The Nordoff-Robbins Music Therapy Monograph Series (Vol. 2). Gilsum, NH: Barcelona.

Aigen, K. (1998). *Paths of development in Nordoff-Robbins Music Therapy.* Phoenixville, PA: Barcelona.

Aigen, K. (1999). The true nature of music-centered music therapy theory. *British Journal of Music Therapy, 13*(2), 77–82.

Aigen, K. (2002/2005). *Playin' in the band: A qualitative study of popular music styles as clinical improvisation.* Gilsum, NH: Barcelona.

Aigen, K. (2005). *Music-centered music therapy.* Gilsum, NH: Barcelona.

Aldridge, D. (1996). *Music therapy research and practice in medicine: From out of the silence*. London: Jessica Kingsley.

Aldridge, D., Gustorff, D., & Neugebauer, L. (1995). A preliminary study of creative music therapy in the treatment of children with developmental delay. *Arts-in-Psychotherapy, 22*(3), 189–205.

Aldridge, G. (2000). Improvisation as an assessment of potential in early Alzheimer's disease. In D. Aldridge (Ed.), *Music therapy in dementia care* (pp. 139–165). London: Jessica Kingsley.

Aldridge, G., & Aldridge, D. (2008). *Melody in music therapy: A therapeutic narrative analysis*. London: Jessica Kingsley.

Ansdell, G. (1995). *Music for life: Aspects of creative music therapy with adult clients*. London: Jessica Kingsley.

Ansdell, G. (1999). Challenging premises. *British Journal of Music Therapy, 13*(2), 72–76.

Ansdell, G. (2002). Community music therapy and the winds of change. *Voices: A World Forum for Music Therapy*. Retrieved from http://www.voices.no/mainissues/Voices2(2)ansdell.html

Brown, S. (1999). Some thoughts on music, therapy, and music therapy. *British Journal of Music Therapy, 13*(2), 63–71.

Bruscia, K. E. (1987). *Improvisational models of music therapy*. Springfield, MO: Charles C. Thomas.

Hadley, S. (1998*). Exploring the relationship between life and work in music therapy: The story of Mary Priestley and Clive Robbins*. Unpublished doctoral dissertation, Temple University, Philadelphia.

Ishizuka, O. (1998). *Between words and music: Creative music therapy as verbal and non-verbal communication with people with dementia*. Unpublished master's thesis, City University, London, U.K. [Online abstract]. Retrieved from http://www.nordoff-robbins.org.uk/html/research.html

Lee, C. (1996). *Music at the edge: The music therapy experiences of a musician with AIDS*. New York: Routledge.

Lee, C. (2003). *The architecture of aesthetic music therapy*. Gilsum, NH: Barcelona.

Maslow, A. (1968). *Toward a psychology of being*. New York: Van Nostrand Reinhold.

Nordoff, P., & Robbins, C. (1977). *Creative music therapy*. New York: John Day.

Nordoff, P., & Robbins, C. (1983). *Music therapy in special education* (2nd ed.). St. Louis, MO: MMB Music.

Nordoff, P., & Robbins, C. (2004). *Therapy in music for handicapped children*. Gilsum, NH: Barcelona.

Nordoff, P., & Robbins, C. (2007). *Creative music therapy: A guide to fostering clinical musicianship* (2nd ed., revised and expanded). Gilsum, NH: Barcelona.

Nordoff-Robbins Center for Music Therapy. (2001a). *The clinical internship*. Retrieved from http://www.nyu.edu/education/music/nrobbins/04pr103certificate.htm

Nordoff-Robbins Center for Music Therapy. (2001b). *Contemporary developments, perspectives, and applications in Nordoff-Robbins Music Therapy*. Retrieved from http://www.nyu.edu/education/music/nrobbins/03developments1.htm

Nordoff-Robbins Center for Music Therapy. (2001c). *History of Nordoff-Robbins Music Therapy*. Retrieved from http://www.nyu.edu/education/music/nrobbins/02history1.htm#history

Nordoff-Robbins Center for Music Therapy. (2001d). *Introduction*. Retrieved from http://www.nyu.edu/education/music/nrobbins/

Nordoff-Robbins Center for Music Therapy. (2001e). *Training programs overview*. Retrieved from http://www.nyu.edu/education/music/nrobbins/04pr1021training.htm

Pavlicevic, M. (1997). *Music therapy in context: Music, meaning, and relationship*. London: Jessica Kingsley.

Pavlicevic, M. (1999). Thoughts, words, and deeds. Harmonies and counterpoints in music therapy theory. *British Journal of Music Therapy, 13*(2), 59–62.

Pavlicevic, M., & Ansdell, G. (2004). *Community music therapy*. London: Jessica Kingsley.

Ritholz, M. S., & Turry, A. (1994). The journey by train: Creative music therapy with a 17-year-old boy. *Music Therapy, 12*(2), 58–87.

Robbins, C. (1993). The creative processes are universal. In M. Heal & T. Wigram (Eds.), *Music therapy in health and education* (pp. 7–25). London: Jessica Kingsley.

Robbins, C. (1997). *What a wonderful song her life sang! An anthology of appreciation for Carol Robbins*. New York: The International Trust for Nordoff-Robbins Music Therapy.

Robbins, C. (2005). *A journey into creative music therapy*. Gilsum, NH: Barcelona

Robbins, C., & Robbins, C. (1980). *Music for the hearing impaired: A resource manual and curriculum guide*. St. Louis, MO: Magnamusic-Baton. [Note: This work is out of print and available only through the Nordoff-Robbins Center for Music Therapy at New York University.]

Robbins, C., & Robbins, C. (Eds.). (1998). *Healing heritage: Paul Nordoff exploring the tonal language of music*. Gilsum, NH: Barcelona.

Robel, K. (1997). *Moving the spirit: The motivational power of music in neurological rehabilitation: Creative music therapy with stroke patients*. Unpublished master's thesis, City University, London, U.K. [Online abstract]. Retrieved from http://www.nordoff-robbins.org.uk/html/research.html

Simpson, F. (2007). *Every note counts: The story of Nordoff-Robbins Music Therapy*. London: James & James.

Streeter, E. (1999). Finding a balance between psychological thinking and musical awareness in music therapy theory: A psychoanalytic perspective. *British Journal of Music Therapy, 13*(1), 5–20.

Turry, A. (1998). Transference and countertransference in Nordoff-Robbins Music Therapy. In K. Bruscia (Ed.), *The dynamics of music psychotherapy* (pp. 161–212). Gilsum, NH: Barcelona.

Turry, A. (2007). *The connection between words and music in music therapy improvisation: An examination of a therapist's method*. Unpublished doctoral dissertation, New York University.

Recommended Additional Readings

Aigen, K. (1995). An aesthetic foundation of clinical theory: An underlying basis of Creative Music Therapy. In C. B. Kenny (Ed.), *Listening, playing, creating: Essays on the power of sound* (pp. 233–257). New York: State University of New York Press.

Brown, S., & Pavlicevic, M. (1996). Clinical improvisation in creative music therapy: Musical aesthetic and the interpersonal dimension. *The Arts in Psychotherapy, 23*(5), 397–406.

Logis, M., & Turry, A. (1999). Singing my way through it: Facing the cancer, darkness and fear. In J. Hibben (Ed.), *Inside music therapy: Client experiences* (pp. 97–117).Gilsum, NH: Barcelona.

Marcus, D., & Turry, A. (2003). Using the Nordoff-Robbins approach to music therapy with adults diagnosed with autism. In D. J. Weiner and L. K. Oxford (Eds.), *Action therapy with families and group: Using creative arts improvisation in clinical practice* (pp. 197–228). Washington, DC: American Psychological Association.

Robarts, J. (1996).Music therapy for children with autism. In C. Trevarthen, K. Aitken, D. Papoudi, & J. Robarts (Eds.), *Children with autism: Diagnosis and intervention to meet their needs* (pp. 134–160). London: Jessica Kingsley.

Robbins, C., & Forinash, M. (1991). A time paradigm: Time as a multilevel phenomenon in music therapy. *Music Therapy, 10*(1), 46–57.

Robbins, C., & Robbins, C. (1991). Creative music therapy in bringing order, change and communicativeness to the life of a brain-injured adolescent. In K. E. Bruscia (Ed.), *Case studies in music therapy* (pp. 231–249). Phoenixville, PA: Barcelona.

Robbins, C., & Robbins, C. (1991). Self-communications in creative music therapy. In K. E. Bruscia (Ed.), *Case studies in music therapy* (pp. 55–72). Phoenixville, PA: Barcelona.

Sorel, S. N. (2005). *Presenting Carly and Elliot: Exploring roles and relationships in a mother-son dyad in Nordoff-Robbins Music Therapy*. Unpublished doctoral dissertation, New York University.

Turry, A., & Marcus, D. (2005). Teamwork: Therapist and cotherapist in the Nordoff-Robbins approach to music therapy. *Music Therapy Perspectives, 23*(1), 53–69.

Recommended Musical Resources

Nordoff, P., & Robbins, C. (1962). *Children's play-songs, first book*. Bryn Mawr, PA: Theodore Presser.

Nordoff, P., & Robbins, C. (1968). *Children's play-songs, second book*. Bryn Mawr, PA: Theodore Presser.

Nordoff, P., & Robbins, C. (1982). *Children's play-songs, third book*. Bryn Mawr, PA: Theodore Presser.

Nordoff, P., & Robbins, C. (1982). *Children's play-songs, fourth book*. Bryn Mawr, PA: Theodore Presser.

Nordoff, P., & Robbins, C. (1982) . *Children's play-songs, fifth book*. Bryn Mawr, PA: Theodore Presser.

Ritholz, M., & Robbins, C. (Eds.). (1999). *Themes for therapy from the Nordoff-Robbins Center for Music Therapy at New York University*. New York: Carl Fischer.

Ritholz, M., & Robbins, C. (Eds.). (2003). *More themes for therapy from the Nordoff-Robbins Center for Music Therapy at New York University*. New York: Carl Fischer.

Robbins, C., & Robbins, C. (1995). *Greetings and goodbyes*. Bryn Mawr, PA: Theodore Presser.

Chapter 7

Psychodynamic Approach to Music Therapy

Connie Isenberg
Frances Smith Goldberg
Janice M. Dvorkin

Introduction

The findings of a recent study on music therapy practice in mental health reveal that 49.2% of psychiatric music therapists who responded reported using a psychodynamic approach, but only 5.7% considered their primary philosophical orientation as psychodynamic (Silverman, 2007). This finding is possibly an artifact of the research methodology, but it does suggest that it is important to address psychodynamic music therapy theory and practice in a way that elucidates theory and illustrates practice.

The nature of music therapy, from both a theoretical and a clinical perspective, has long been the subject of discussion and debate. Two fundamental questions arise: Does music therapy depend upon the music for its therapeutic essence, or does the therapy unfold within the relationship between the therapist and the patient? This question, which has particular relevance for psychodynamic music therapy, was addressed as early as 1968 by Schneider, Unkefer, and Gaston in their introduction to E. Thayer Gaston's book *Music in Therapy*, in which they described three stages of development in the field. During the first stage, emphasis was placed on the importance of music to the exclusion of the therapeutic relationship; in the second, the emphasis was reversed, with a focus that was almost exclusively on the therapeutic relationship; and in the third stage, a balance between the two extremes was attempted. This debate regarding the role of music still persists but has shifted in emphasis. Whereas in the third stage it was recognized that both the music and the therapist were essential components of the process, current concerns focus more specifically on the relative importance of music versus words (e.g., Erkkilä, 2004).

The second question asks whether music therapy has its own independent theoretical framework, or is it dependent upon extant theories? Both Ruud (1980) and Wheeler (1981, 1983,

1987) addressed this question. Ruud looked at a variety of theories, including psychoanalytic theory, to explore their contribution to the understanding and practice of music therapy. He described the psychodynamic meaning and functions of music as articulated by psychoanalytic theorists. Wheeler also explored the relationship between music therapy and a variety of psychotherapy theories, ranging from the behavioral to the psychodynamic. Both Ruud and Wheeler alluded to the unique nature of music therapy but expressed the importance of remaining open to existing theoretical models. Stressing that theories of music therapy need to be based upon psychological theories, Ruud nonetheless identified the examination of the relationship between man and music as being the unique contribution of music therapy to the understanding of human beings. Wheeler cited two benefits of relying on psychotherapeutic theories, in that these theories provide a conceptual map for the clinical work and may also serve to enhance the status of the profession within the mental health community. In support of Wheeler's view, it is of note that music remains an object of interest for psychoanalysts to this day. Some psychoanalysts focus on the elucidation of musical works through a psychoanalytic lens (e.g., Rusbridger, 2008); others focus on the psychic functions of music (e.g., Lipson, 2006; Stein, 2004). Lecourt (2004), a French music therapist and psychoanalyst, looked at the psychic functions of music for the individual and group and explored music therapy as psychoanalytic work. This second fundamental question of newly constructed music-based theories (e.g., Aigen, 1995; Kenny, 1989) versus borrowed theoretical frameworks has also not been resolved. There is, nonetheless, important work being done in this area. Erkkilä (2004) and Salmon (2008) emphasized the commonalities between music therapy and psychodynamic psychotherapy, with Salmon identifying five common elements: listening, time, affect, mourning, and creativity/play. Lecourt, mentioned above, and Ahonen-Eerikainen (2007), rather than identifying similarities and differences, simply defined music therapy as a form of psychodynamic therapy, and Metzner (2004) provided arguments for viewing receptive music therapy from a psychoanalytic perspective. This chapter focuses on the application and adaptation of a borrowed theoretical framework, that is, the psychodynamic one, to the practice of music therapy.

As stated above, there has been a shift over time in the debate regarding the role of music versus the role of the relationship in music psychotherapy. Bruscia (1998c) contributed to the current debate regarding the role of music by looking at the relative importance attributed to the musical process versus the verbal process within the therapeutic context. It is the verbal process that supplants the earlier references to the relationship. He described four levels of engagement used in music psychotherapy. These fall on a continuum from the exclusively musical to the exclusively verbal:

- Music as psychotherapy: The therapeutic issue is accessed, worked through, and resolved through creating or listening to music, with no need for or use of verbal discourse.
- Music-centered psychotherapy: The therapeutic issue is accessed, worked through, and resolved through creating or listening to music; verbal discourse is used to guide, interpret, or enhance the music experience and its relevance to the client and therapeutic process.
- Music in psychotherapy: The therapeutic issue is accessed, worked through, and resolved through both musical and verbal experiences, occurring either alternately or simultaneously. Music is used for its specific and unique qualities and is germane to the

therapeutic issue and its treatment; words are used to identify and consolidate insights gained during the process.

• Verbal psychotherapy with music: The therapeutic issue is accessed, worked through, and resolved primarily through verbal discourse. Music experiences may be used in tandem to facilitate or enrich the discussion, but are not considered germane to the therapeutic issue or treatment of it. (Bruscia, 1998c, p. 2)

The first two levels of engagement, music as psychotherapy and music-centered psychotherapy, are further described as transformative music psychotherapy because these represent approaches in which the music experience itself is considered to be the agent of change. In contrast, the next two levels of engagement, that is, music in psychotherapy and verbal psychotherapy with music, are referred to as insight music psychotherapy. Insight music therapy refers to those approaches in which the verbal exchange rather than the musical experience is viewed as the agent of change. As Bruscia (1998a) stated, "It is the verbally mediated awareness gained as the result of the music experience that leads to change" (p. 214).

Adapting Wolberg's (1977) psychotherapy typology to music therapy, Wheeler (1983) identified three levels of music therapy: music therapy as activity therapy, insight music therapy with re-educative goals, and insight music therapy with reconstructive goals. At both levels of insight music therapy as defined by Wheeler, the "unique nonverbal advantages of music," to use Bruscia's words (1998a, p. 214), and the insight-enhancing qualities of verbal communication are fully exploited. The therapist pays attention to transference/countertransference reactions and to defenses. The differences between these two levels are related to the temporal and the topographic components, in other words, the targeted time frame and the levels of consciousness addressed. When working with re-educative goals, the therapist focuses on the here-and-now and restricts interpretations to the patient's conscious and preconscious material. With reconstructive goals, the focus is expanded to include the past, and unconscious material becomes the object of the therapist's active intervention. Despite their differences, both insight levels of music therapy can be classified as psychodynamically based.

Before looking directly at the development of psychodynamic music therapy, let us now turn our attention to a brief outline of the history and development of psychodynamic theory so that we can better understand how it informs the theory and practice of psychodynamic music therapy.

History and Development of Psychodynamic Theory

In this section, we will briefly present psychodynamic theory, from its origins in Freudian psychoanalytic theory, through its developments in object relations theory, self psychology, and, most recently, intersubjective theory. Several terms are commonly used to label the forms of psychotherapy described by these theories: *psychoanalytic psychotherapy, psychodynamic psychotherapy,* and *insight-oriented psychotherapy.* These terms are considered interchangeable for our purposes and all refer to clinical practices that have evolved from classical psychoanalysis as developed by Sigmund Freud.

It is important to note that, whereas some disciples and proponents of Freud modified his theory and can loosely be perceived as falling within a "Freudian line" of theorists, others can be better characterized as dissenters who eventually diverged sharply from his approach, developing their own theory and practice. Jung was such a dissenter. Analytical psychology, developed by Jung, diverged from its Freudian origins in both content and form and forged its own distinct identity.[1] While recognizing the importance of Jungian theory within music therapy, we do not elaborate upon it in this section. Illustrations of the use of Jungian concepts within the music psychotherapeutic process can, however, be found in the clinical applications section of this chapter.

Freudian Theory

Freudian theory is a meta-psychological theory, which provides us with a comprehensive framework for understanding mental life. It describes psychic structures and systems of consciousness from a developmental perspective. It can be viewed as a theory of meaning upon which an interpretive discipline is based. Inherent to Freudian theory is the belief that mental health can be achieved by acquiring an understanding of why the problem symptoms exist and from where they originate. In other words, it is believed that the patient's acquisition of insight into the meaning and genetic roots of symptoms, with the help of the therapist's interpretations, can be curative.

Freudian theory is vast, and so we will highlight several key concepts. Fundamental to Freudian theory is the concept of *drives*. Freud believed that humans are motivated by two instinctual drives—aggressive and libidinal. These drives can be viewed as opposite tendencies, struggling against each other for control of mental life. The struggle of opposing forces inherent to Freudian theory defines it as a *conflict theory*. Conflict can also express itself among the structures of the psychical apparatus described by Freud, that is, the id, the ego and the superego. For example, physical symptoms that are not accounted for medically could be an expression of overwhelming anxiety resulting from an internal conflict between these three structures of mental organization. A defining characteristic of Freudian theory and wider psychodynamic theory is that internal conflict functions on an *unconscious* level.

Let us look at the mental structures of *id*, *ego*, and *superego* from a developmental perspective. A child is born in a diffuse psychic state, a nondifferentiated id state. In this state, mental functioning is dominated by the *pleasure principle* and is focused on the satisfaction of basic needs, such as hunger and thirst. The goal of the pleasure principle is immediate gratification of the drives, as evidenced by the infant's needs. At approximately 2 years of age, the child's ego becomes differentiated from the id in reaction to realistic demands to contain or frustrate the id impulses. As the ego struggles to tame id impulses, the pleasure principle is supplanted by the *reality principle*. The reality principle takes the conditions of the external world into consideration. Inherent to this principle is an implication that greater satisfaction can be obtained through postponement than by striving for immediate gratification of needs. At approximately 4 years of age, the superego develops as an internalization of the parents' moral standards and

> sets up and maintains an intricate system of ideals and values, prohibitions and commands (the conscience). It observes and evaluates the self, compares it with the ideal and either criticizes,

---

[1] Readings on Jungian analytical psychology are found on the recommended reading list.

reproaches and punishes, leading to a variety of painful affects, or praises and rewards, thereby raising self esteem. (Moore & Fine, 1990, p. 189)

The ego functions to achieve a balance between the impulsive demands of the id, the moral pressures of the superego, and the demands of reality.

Another aspect of classical psychodynamic theory that we will touch upon is the *psychosexual stage theory* of child development. Freud's theory maintains there are five stages of psychosexual development, each stage related to the parts of the body that become the focus of libidinal drives. The stages are, in order: oral, anal, phallic, latency, and genital. As one goes through the stages, remnants of previous stages are always present. When these are present to an excessive degree, this is referred to as *fixation*. The genital stage is considered to occur following the transformations of puberty.

The goal of therapy in this classical model is to bring the internal conflicts to consciousness, or, in other words, to render the unconscious conscious. Some ways to bring the unconscious to consciousness are through the reporting of dreams, screen memories (defensive compromise memories in which insignificant details are remembered with clarity and imbued with importance), and *free association* (reporting all thoughts occurring to the person during the therapy session). All verbalizations are explored and analyzed, as are nonverbal behaviors. Within the context of psychodynamic music therapy, music preferences and musical expression can also be considered a way to bring unconscious feelings to consciousness. Examples can include the unconscious humming of a musical selection (Diaz de Chumaceiro, 1998), a desire to listen to a specific piece of music, free associative singing (Austin, 1996), and instrumental improvisation (Ahonen-Eerikainen, 2004).

An unconscious hesitancy or refusal to engage in free association during therapy is considered to be a *resistance* or an impediment to the therapeutic process. According to Freud, the major reason for resistance is to avoid the anxiety generated by the threat of the failure of repression. *Repression* refers to the unconscious "forgetting" of anxiety-provoking ideational and perceptual content, thereby keeping it out of the conscious mind. *Defense mechanisms* are unconscious coping mechanisms employed to ward off anxiety and in this way function in the service of resistance. They must, therefore, be analyzed within the context of therapy. (Refer to Austin & Dvorkin, 1998, for examples of resistance in music therapy.)

In order to accomplish the goal of therapy, the therapist must maintain as much *neutrality* as possible. In this way, the patient's attitude towards the therapist is not triggered by the person of the therapist per se, but rather reflects the patient's projections and displacements on to the therapist from significant people in the patient's past. These can include parents, siblings, and others. The patient's perceptions of the therapist are therefore distortions of reality. This process is called *transference* and is encouraged through the neutrality of the therapist. Transference is considered the hallmark of psychodynamic psychotherapy. If the therapist's reaction to the patient is based on his or her own projections or displacements, this is referred to as *countertransference*, or the therapist's transference. Whereas Freud had originally considered countertransference an obstacle and something to be worked through, the understanding of the concept of countertransference has evolved. Paula Heimann (1950) was the first to recognize the importance of countertransference, that is, the therapist's emotional response to the patient, as a therapeutic tool. The concept of countertransference is currently the focus of much attention in the music therapy literature. A few examples follow. Using a qualitative research approach,

Dillard (2006) examined the impact of musical countertransference on the therapist's understanding of patients and on treatment. Marom (2008) elaborates upon the complicated countertransference reactions triggered by patients in hospice care and underlines how important it is for the therapist to become aware of these countertransference reactions. Scheiby (2005) describes how musical improvisation reflects both the patient's transference and the therapist's countertransference. (For further examples, refer to Dvorkin & Erlund, 2003.)

Object Relations Theory

Object Relations theory can be viewed as an extension of Freudian theory. While maintaining many of the same basic concepts, Object Relations theory is distinguished from Freudian theory in that the therapeutic focus is shifted away from drive and intrapsychic conflict to an interpersonal component. In other words, the focus is on the patient's *relational* problems. It is through the understanding of the patient's internalized objects as expressed toward the therapist that the therapeutic work can occur. It is important to note that, in the language of psychodynamic theory, objects refer to people. *Internal objects* refer to the internalized representation of the external object. We all create within ourselves an internalized image of our significant others. It is these images that we then project on to others. The goal of Object Relations psychodynamic therapy is to help the patient become aware of how internalized object relations are repeated in current external relationships and are at the source of current interpersonal difficulties. The therapist attempts to provide a reparative experience by focusing on unmet developmental needs, thereby promoting the formation of good object relationships.

In the British school of Object Relations, from Melanie Klein to D. W. Winnicott, the focus of therapy is on developing a way to work psychodynamically with people who have difficulty forming satisfactory relationships. The explanatory theory shifts from a conflict theory to a *deficiency theory*. Symptoms are viewed as resulting from an arrest in development due to the initial caretaker's inability to meet the infant's psychological needs. The American school of Object Relations, including Kernberg, Mahler, and Masterson, focuses on the way in which therapeutic intervention results in an ameliorated separation/individuation experience (Detrick & Detrick, 1989).

The therapist's role, in this model of therapy, is to understand the patient's earliest relationship by encouraging the development of the *transference*. The goal is to help the patient experience a "good enough" relationship with a mother-substitute, thereby changing the patient's perception of relationships. This effect is often achieved through the use of the therapist's *holding* or *containment* of the patient's concerns, thoughts, and feelings. In psychodynamic music therapy, this may be expressed through the therapist's ability to withstand the patient's intense emotional musical expression, be it in the form of loud anger or inconsolable grief, without being destroyed. This is often a new experience for the patient. A good-enough newly internalized object may now lead to a sense of security and belonging, which in turn may lead to a basic sense of trust. The patient may then be able to continue through the stages of psychosocial development. (For additional examples, see the following case studies: Inada, 2007; Jahn-Langenberg, 2003; Nolan, 2003; Robarts, 2003.)

The concept of a transitional object was developed by D. W. Winnicott (1971) to describe a process whereby an inanimate object can serve as a substitute for the soothing effect of the mother, thereby facilitating separation from the caretaker. A song can function as a transitional object, thereby being used as a self-soothing device.

Self Psychology

Self psychology is the next development in psychodynamic therapy. This theory, developed by Heinz Kohut, can be viewed as a *deprivation* model, in that the patient has an insufficiently developed self because of the limitations of the self-object experiences with significant others in the early stages of life. The person, therefore, spends his or her life trying to obtain these essential experiences from others.

The different types of *self-object experiences* include mirroring self-objects, which provide confirmation for the child's innate sense of vigor, greatness, and perfection; idealized self-objects, which are made available to the child as emanating from images of calmness, infallibility, and omnipotence, with which the child can merge; alter-ego self-objects, which are needed to become models and provide experiences of likeness that sustain the self and stimulate the potential for learning; and adversarial self-objects, which are needed for healthy assertiveness vis-à-vis the caregiver without fear of impairing the self-object relationship (Wolf, 1988).

Through the use of *empathy*, the therapist is able to provide the self-object relationships required. Since the patient's sense of self is built through the eyes of others, the therapist is encouraged to communicate understanding through a reflection of what the patient expresses. Musically, the therapist's responses need to be supportive and reflective. Mirroring is also an essential component of the musical process. The therapist needs to learn how to interpret the music, whether chosen or improvised, as well as to compare the music from session to session so as to follow the therapy process through the music. (For examples of reflection and interpretation, refer to Pavlicevic, 1997; for mirroring, refer to Austin, 1991.)

Intersubjective Theory

The most recent extension of psychodynamic theory incorporates the concept of intersubjectivity within the analytic relationship. Stolorow, Brandschaft, and Atwood (1987) suggested that psychodynamic investigation "is always from a perspective within a subjective world (the patient's or the analyst's); it is always empathic or introspective" (p. 5). They define psychodynamic understanding "as an intersubjective process involving a dialogue between two personal universes" (p. 7). They went on to say that "the reality that crystallizes in the course of . . . treatment is an intersubjective reality" (p. 7).

A notion of objectivity or neutrality as the purview of the therapist has no place within this conceptualization of the patient-therapist relationship. This theory posits that therapeutic abstinence, as a clinical principle, that is, the absence of gratification of patients' needs, is inimical to therapeutic change. Rather than remaining neutral, therapists should monitor what in their behavior will facilitate the transformation of the patient's subjective world. According to Stolorow et al. (1987), the therapeutic stance that is required is one of "*sustained empathic inquiry*" (p. 10), which brings the intersubjective relationship between the therapist and patient to the forefront. The change process is not, therefore, exclusively internal to the patient, but is believed to occur within a specific intersubjective system.

Within this framework, the patient's experience of the therapeutic exchange is seen as being codetermined by the activities of both participants. The therapist needs, therefore, to be particularly careful about the degree and form of his or her reactions to the behaviors and expressions of the patient. Which aspects of intervention need special attention within the context of psychodynamic music therapy? In the Bonny Method of Guided Imagery and Music (BMGIM), the selection of music for the session as well as the therapist's comments made during the interactive dialogue in the music experience require specific attention. Improvisationally, the therapist needs to attend to the more personal musical responses in reaction to those of the patient. The notion inherent to Intersubjective theory, that the patient's experience is codetermined by the therapist, lends itself to psychodynamic music therapy. The co-creative possibilities of improvisational music therapy as they unfold within the context of a psychodynamic framework are discussed by Turry (1998).

Current Literature of Psychodynamic Music Therapy

Having reviewed the major schools of psychodynamic thought, let us now turn our attention back to the development of psychodynamic music therapy. Not so long ago, when we evoked the term *psychodynamic music therapy,* the names that sprang to mind were few in number. Certainly, Florence Tyson (1965, 1981) was an early American proponent of the use of a music therapy psychodynamic orientation, as was Juliette Alvin (1975) in England. It was Mary Priestley's book *Music Therapy in Action* (1975), however, that seemed to capture the attention of a wide number of music therapists. Her model of psychodynamic music therapy known as Analytical Music Therapy has taken hold and has been further developed by many clinicians and theoreticians in her home country, England, throughout Europe, and more recently in North America. Whereas psychodynamic music therapy has had strong footholds in various parts of Europe (we need only think of Edith Lecourt [1993, 1994] in France and Johannes Th. Eschen in Germany), the North American developments are more recent.

We are currently witnessing a burgeoning interest in psychodynamic music therapy, so it is unusual these days to find even an introductory textbook or handbook that does not make reference to psychodynamic music therapy (e.g., Darnley-Smith, & Patey, 2003; Schmidt-Peters, 2000). A proliferation of literature addresses psychodynamic music therapy, with some books dealing exclusively with psychodynamic approaches, while others include other approaches as well. Bruscia (1998b), Eschen (2002), and Hadley (2003) have provided us with examples of the former. Bruscia devoted an entire book to the dynamics of the music psychotherapeutic relationship, with a specific emphasis on transference-countertransference phenomena, and Hadley provided us with a collection of case studies in psychodynamic music therapy. In both of these books, a wide variety of psychodynamic music therapy approaches is represented. Eschen, in contrast, has gathered writings on one specific approach, Analytical Music Therapy (see below), and Ahonen-Eerikäinen (2007) has presented a psychodynamic group music psychotherapeutic process, which she entitles Group Analytic Music Therapy. Pavlicevic (1997, 1999) reflected on the meaning of psychodynamic concepts within the context of psychodynamic music therapy and paid particular attention to Winnicott's theory. Wigram and De Backer (1999), although providing us with writings on a variety of clinical approaches within psychiatry, included several chapters on psychodynamic approaches. The widespread interest in and adherence to a psychodynamic music therapy framework is reflected clearly in the countries represented by the authors contributing to Hadley's (2003) book of case studies. One Australian, 11 Europeans (Belgium, Denmark, France, Germany, and Italy), 4 British, 1 Israeli, and 8 Americans authored chapters. Johannes Eschen's (2002) book on analytical music therapy reflects the same widespread impact of psychodynamic music therapy, the authors representing European countries, the United States, and Canada.

The psychodynamic theories reflected in psychodynamic music therapy practice abound. Wigram, Pedersen, and Bonde (2002) cited the following theorists as having had the most influence on psychodynamic music therapy in Europe: Freud, Jung, Klein, Winnicott, Mahler, Kohut, and Stern (psychology of intersubjectivity). It is no different on the other side of the ocean. Having already looked at the development of many of these models, we will use the case material below to elucidate the application of some of these theories within the context of psychodynamic music therapy. We will, however, first take a brief look at one form of psychodynamic music therapy, that is, Analytical Music Therapy.

Analytical Music Therapy

What is Analytical Music Therapy? Mary Priestley described this improvisational form of music therapy as a way of exploring the patient's unconscious through the use of musical and verbal expression (Eschen, 2002; Priestley, 1975, 1994). The relationship that develops between the therapist and the patient, as it unfolds through transferential and countertransferential reactions, is understood to be the locus of therapeutic action. Although derived from Kleinian psychoanalysis, Priestly insisted upon the distinctions. In her words, "Analytical Music Therapy was born out of psychoanalysis, but it is very different from psychoanalysis" (Priestley & Eschen, 2002, p. 11). She highlighted that, when the patient and the therapist play together, there is a real shared experience, a real gratification of a desire for closeness. Unlike the rule of abstinence in psychoanalysis, this shared music may symbolically represent the satisfaction of more primitive or libidinal desires (Priestley, 1975). She stressed the difference between the verbal relationship and the musical one. "In the music . . . we are closer and more open about our response to the client's feelings. Together we are creating something that has never been there before, and together we listen to the playback" (Priestley & Eschen, 2002, p. 13). She believed that the music therapist's improvisational response must reflect his or her personhood to be effective. Employing a historical reconstructive case study methodology, Eyre (2007) has recently provided us with the first comprehensive qualitative study of an Analytical Music Therapy process conducted by Mary Priestley. Eyre examined the manifestations of change as reflected in images, life changes, and musical expression, and interpreted the findings from a psychodynamic perspective.

Training

Intrinsic to Priestley's model is a training program for analytic music therapists, which involves a personal therapeutic process. Freud (1926/2001) emphasized the analyst's responsibility "to make himself capable, by a deep-going analysis of his own, of the unprejudiced reception of the analytic material" (p. 220). In this way, he insisted upon the training analysis as an essential prerequisite to the practice of analysis. Both Priestley (1994) and Helen Bonny

(2002) have prescribed a personal therapeutic process within their respective approaches as a prerequisite for practice. Within Priestley's model, the training consists of two stages. In the first stage, the student engages in an individual analytical music therapy process with a trained analytical music therapist. In the Bonny Method of Guided Imagery and Music (BMGIM), the obligatory personal therapy component within the training process consists of a series of individual BMGIM sessions with a trained BMGIM therapist. In both approaches, this allows for the student's own exploration of inner life using the same therapeutic form that that is being learned. In other words, the student can begin to learn about the approach from the inside. In the second stage of Analytical Music Therapy training, Intertherapy, two students engage in a process with one teacher who serves as supervisor. The students change roles, alternating between therapist and patient. During these sessions, the students do not role play but deal with their own life issues. According to Priestley, they focus on verbal language, body language, and musical language. It is to be noted that both of these models can be viewed as specializations for trained music therapists.

Psychodynamic Language Versus Psychodynamic Process

In contrast with Priestley, Alvin (1975) used the terms of psychodynamic therapy, but not the words related to the therapeutic relationship. In describing the psychological effects of music, as she understands them expressed in her free improvisation technique, she stated:

> Music works at id, ego, and superego levels. It can stir up or express primitive instincts and even help to let them loose—it can help to strengthen the ego, release and control the emotions at the same time . . . it can sublimate certain emotions, satisfy the desire for perfection . . . (p. 77)

She went on to say that "music can be a projective means. It creates an emotional state in which the patient is ready to recall his problems, his obsessions, and his inhibitions and to face them (p. 134). "The breaking up of defenses is one of the most generally accepted effects of music in psychotherapy. Music can become a bridge between reality and the unreal world in which the patient is isolated or takes refuge" (p. 141). Whereas she very coherently and elaborately described the relationship of the patient to the music in psychodynamic terms, her description of the relationship between the patient and the therapist in psychodynamic terms is quite limited.

Psychodynamic Thought in Psychodynamic Music Therapy

Having reviewed the major schools of psychodynamic thought, let us now reflect on how these can be useful to us as psychodynamic music therapy clinicians. We must ask ourselves the following questions regarding each theoretical framework: How does it allow us to understand the patient's inner world? How does it allow us to understand the expression of this inner world within the unfolding therapeutic process? How does it allow us to understand the musical process within the therapeutic context? The importance of these questions becomes clearer once we realize that there is no direct correspondence between a specific music therapy approach or technique and a specific conceptual framework. It is the therapist's clinical thought, that is, the therapist's understanding of the unfolding therapeutic process rather than his or her specific therapeutic action, that is determined by the conceptual framework. The corollary is that we can identify a music psychotherapeutic orientation via the therapist's clinical thought rather than through therapeutic action. Psychodynamic music therapists use a variety of music therapy approaches, such as vocal improvisation (e.g., Austin, 1999) and instrumental improvisation (e.g., Nolan, 1994), song writing, patient-selected music, music imagery, and the Bonny Method of Guided Imagery and Music (e.g., Goldberg, 2000). Music therapists who do not consider themselves psychodynamic therapists use some of these same approaches. Through simple observation, we cannot necessarily distinguish between BMGIM that is being conceptualized as a transpersonal process and BMGIM that is being conceptualized as a psychodynamic process. Nor can we always distinguish between improvisational techniques that are being used within a psychodynamic framework and the same techniques being used within another framework. Since clinical thought is expressed through a clinical vocabulary or language (Isenberg-Grzeda, 1989, 1998), we are able to identify the commonly held concepts that underlie psychodynamic music therapy.

What are some of the extra-musical commonly held concepts?

- The concept of the *unconscious*, that is, a system of consciousness of which we are unaware but that has a tremendous influence on our behavior, thoughts, and feelings. Inherent to this concept is the notion that the past influences the present.
- The concept of the *transference* (*countertransference*) is the hallmark of psychodynamic theory. It refers to the way in which old relationships and patterns are repeated in the therapeutic setting and highlights how central the relationship is to the change process. Change occurs through the working through of the transference, that is, through the working through of the unconscious relationship with the therapist. The relationship with the therapist is, therefore, fundamental to the treatment process. Countertransference refers to the therapist's reactions to the patient.
- The concepts of *defenses* and *resistance* help us to understand that, as much as our patients strive to change, the change process is fraught with obstacles. It is among the therapist's functions to help the patient overcome resistance.
- Although the concept of verbally-mediated *insight* is not universally accepted within psychodynamic music therapy, there is an implicit recognition of the importance of increased *awareness* and understanding.
- Although the concept of *abstinence*, that is, the nongratification of needs by the therapist, has been put into question within the intersubjective framework, a notion of some degree of therapist *neutrality* is still commonly supported.
- A concept that seeks to explain the origin of the pathology and its symptoms is common to all. The original explanatory concept was that of unconscious *conflict* and is identified most strongly with Freud. Another explanatory concept is that of *deficiency* and is identified most strongly with Winnicott and Kohut. It should be noted that the therapist's belief in one or the other of these concepts, or both, will have a direct impact on the therapeutic work.

What are some of the music-related commonly held concepts?

- Music can serve as a form of free association (Freud-based).
- Music can help make the unconscious conscious (Freud-based).
- Music can receive split-off parts of the self or the other, in other words, can receive projections (Klein-based).
- Music can serve as a transitional object (Winnicott-based).
- Music can serve as a container or a holding environment (Bion-based).
- Music can serve as a mirror (Kohut-based).
- Music can hold transference, countertransference and intersubjective responses (Freud-, Stern-, Stolorow and Atwood-based).

Clinical Applications of Psychodynamic Music Therapy

In this section we will present clinical examples using different music therapy approaches, as well as different frames for understanding the work. They will help to clarify how the above-mentioned concepts, both musical and extra-musical, unfold within the clinical context. Four clinical vignettes and one brief therapy case will illustrate the variety of music therapy approaches employed by psychodynamic music therapists; psychodynamic concepts; the relative use of music versus words in the therapeutic process; and the interaction of the triadic relationship of music, client, and therapist (Summer, 1998). (One of the authors, Goldberg, is the music therapist in the first and third clinical vignettes and the brief case study, with the second and fourth vignettes taken from other sources.)

First Clinical Vignette

Jim

Music therapy approaches: Music Imagery
                             Client-selected music

Psychodynamic concepts: Making the unconscious conscious
                           "Working through" an issue through music experiences

Jim was a 49-year-old white, married, successful businessman and father of three children. He was very engaging, intelligent, and articulate. He was engaged in a long-term therapy process with me that consisted primarily of the Bonny Method of Guided Imagery and Music (BMGIM), through which we had accessed and worked through several issues. The music therapy approach in this clinical vignette, however, is client-selected music used in a Music Imagery session.

Jim's current preoccupation had to do with his difficulties interacting with colleagues and clients. He was working on his difficulty tolerating any degree of criticism directed toward him or his ideas. He said he just got lost in the conversation when he felt some judgment of him by others, and he wanted to overcome this as it had serious ramifications for him at work. He realized he missed important communications from others when this happened. We had already discovered through his BMGIM sessions that the current difficulty was related to his anger as well as anger from others and that this stemmed from his father yelling at him and his mother when he was a child.

Jim brought Jimi Hendrix's Woodstock performance of the "Star Spangled Banner" to this session as a representation of anger. We decided to use it for a Music Imagery session rather than BMGIM, because the music is too chaotic for BMGIM and also because he said he had never been able to tolerate listening to it all the way through.

Music Imagery is a focused music psychotherapy approach that may take many forms where one of a variety of genres of music is used to support imagery. It can be very directive or nondirective, may include a verbal dialogue between the client and the therapist during the music, and may involve drawing or writing during or after the music experience. The duration of the music experience is, on average, 5 to 15 minutes, and the client sits in a chair while experiencing the music. Most often the session begins with a very specific focus agreed on by the client and the therapist. The therapist may describe the focus using the client's own words as the music begins, or the client may hold the focus on his or her own, as in this vignette. Music Imagery may be used for all three of Wheeler's (1983) levels of therapy: supportive, re-educative, or reconstructive.

We did not engage in a verbal dialogue during the music. Jim was assured that he could open his eyes at any point if it became too overwhelming for him. Also, since he was sitting within arm's length of the stereo equipment, he could turn off the music himself or ask me to do so at any time. The solo electric guitar begins in a rather organized way, with improvised music; however, it gradually deteriorates into chaotic turmoil with no recognizable rhythm, structure, or tonality with a lot of dissonance. There is a great deal of induced electronic feedback and distortion of the sound. When the melody becomes recognizable, there are electronic imitations of "bombs bursting in air" as well. The music feels very aggressive to me.

The first thing Jim said after the music ended was, "This is only the second time in history that this has ever happened." He talked about Moses and the burning bush that was not consumed by fire. The image this music evoked in him was from a BMGIM session a few weeks prior to this session, where he saw a volcano spewing molten lava. This time he was standing in the fire inside the crater of the volcano, but was not consumed by the fire. He said it was frightening, but he decided he needed to stay with it to find out what would happen. He was amazed that he was not even burned, much less consumed. His immediate understanding was that he could tolerate others' anger as well as his own without being "burned." This session had a transforming impact on him, and he reported several instances over the next few months where he would have gone into confusion in the past, but did not. He felt fully free of his fear of anger. He felt he came out of that session a changed man.

Reflection

This session also gave me insight into Jim's experience when faced with criticism or anger. The music was undoubtedly an apt metaphor for his experience of confusion, so close to his experience that prior to this session he could not listen to the music all the way to the end. This session came after many months of therapy and is an example of working through the issue during the music experience. The talking after the session was only to report and validate his experience of withstanding the volcano of anger.

Second Clinical Vignette

Maria

Music therapy approach: Improvisation

Psychodynamic concepts: Making the unconscious conscious
                            "Working through" an issue through music and verbal
                                experiences
                            Music receives the split-off parts of self and other

Margareta Wärja (1994) reported her metaphorical improvisation work with Maria from a Jungian analytical psychology perspective.

Maria, a 45-year-old woman in treatment for depression, came to the session with the following dream: "I dreamt that I was a tree standing stuck in a barren landscape. The wind carried some birds that teased and laughed at me and said that I was doomed to stay there, and that I was not as free as they were." I suggested that Maria pick some instruments to represent the tree and begin to play how the tree feels and what kind of life the tree has. She chose a wood block and a soft bass drum. She played the wood block without resonance, which made the sound dead and hollow. A steady and solid beat from the bass drum was audible underneath the arid and empty sound of the wood block. It made me think of a heart pulsating with life. It was striking how steady and grounded the bass drum was, which pointed toward a strength that Maria had repressed. Next, she made up "the bird teasing tune," an improvisation of cutting, sneering, and squeaking bells and a synthesizer that seemed to score and ridicule her. Both improvisations were recorded and, as we listened to this music over several sessions and talked about it, Maria began to hear what her music wanted to tell her. We also continued the music-making process by playing together and exploring the tree and the birds more fully. Slowly, Maria came to understand how both the tree and the birds were parts of herself that were fighting inside her. For quite a long time, she had seen the birds as her co-workers, who were complaining that she didn't work hard enough, and her mother who was never satisfied. She realized that she herself had internalized these voices and had allowed them to continue to pester her. This had kept her in a victim role and prevented her from becoming responsible for her own life. After continued work in therapy, Maria was able to accept and begin to use her strengths that the "tree drum," that is, the Self had presented to her. (Wärja, 1994, p. 78, used with permission)

Reflection

In Jungian analytical psychology, the Self is one of the principle archetypes (an essential and universal aspect of humanity that is seen in various images that emerge in myths, dreams, music, and other forms of creative expression (Austin, 1996). The Self has purpose and direction and its function is to guide the person toward wholeness. It is also seen as the aspect of the person that brings images and dreams in the service of becoming more whole. Maria's dream brought a healthy part of herself that had been split off from consciousness through the introjection of the voices of her complaining mother and co-workers. However, Maria could not recognize these voices as coming from herself until she engaged in metaphoric improvisation and brought it to consciousness, thus allowing her to release the victim role and be more in control of her life.

Third Clinical Vignette

Elinor

Music therapy approach:	BMGIM
	Improvisation
	Music Imagery
Psychodynamic concepts:	Making the unconscious conscious
	Accessing, "working through" and resolving an issue through music experiences
	"Working through" defenses
	Uncovering and releasing repressed feelings
	Music serves as a container or holding environment

Elinor was a 26-year-old single, white medical resident who came to me for help in separating from her mother and dealing with the attendant guilt. The precipitating event was her mother's suicide attempt. Elinor had moved to this city from the Midwest to begin her residency just 3 weeks prior to our meeting. Elinor presented as an intelligent and articulate young woman. She was very distressed about her mother but did not want to leave her residency to return home. Her mother was chronically suicidal. Elinor, as the youngest of four children, two sisters and one brother, felt very responsible for her divorced mother, since the divorce came when she was 10 years old, and her siblings, who were all several years older than she, had already moved out of the house. She always hurried home from school to make sure her mother was all right. She felt that her mother's current attempt was a manipulative effort to get her to move back home. However, she felt very torn between her feelings of responsibility toward her mother and her quest for her own life.

The two sessions reported here came toward the end of a 2-year therapy process that consisted primarily of BMGIM, supplemented by art and improvisational music. The first of these sessions was a BMGIM session using the music of Wagner, Hansen, Elgar, and Mahler. Elinor found herself wandering aimlessly in a desert. She came to a hill and began to climb. As she climbed, she said the hill was becoming gelatinous and was difficult to climb. After struggling to the top, she slid down the other side, landing in the sand. She was distressed to find that the gelatinous substance was stuck to her body and she could not get it all off. She decided to continue walking and felt that she had direction now, although she still didn't know where she was going. She came to an oasis where a familiar Wise Woman was waiting for her. The Wise Woman cleaned her off and held her. She felt comforted.

The following week Elinor came to the session very upset. She was in touch with what that imagery meant to her: nobody was there to catch her and hold her when she was born. I asked her if she could draw what she was feeling. She used a black oil pastel and vigorously made sharp marks across the paper. She very soon filled the paper with heavy black marks using her whole body in her effort to portray her feelings. I placed a djembe (African drum) in front of her, and she immediately started drumming. Again, she used her whole body, beating loud, irregular rhythms. I supported her with a large plains drum and encouraged her by mirroring her drumming. Her drumming became more and more frenzied as she finally allowed herself to release the repressed anger and hurt. She then collapsed into deep sobs. I supported her crying with a very soft humming. My image was of a small baby.

When the tears subsided, I asked if she would like to put her feelings on paper again. She drew soft pastel colors in a swirling pattern over the entire paper. She expressed great relief and said the colors felt comforting. I then asked her to close her eyes for music imaging. To the strains of Elgar's "Sospiri," I directed her to allow herself to go into her drawing and feel the softness and the comfort of the colors. We were both silent through the 5 minutes of this lovely, slow, piece that to me feels nourishing. At the end of the music, she reported that she had felt the softness of the colors on her skin and felt truly held. She left the session feeling free and renewed. Elinor's therapy came to an end a few weeks after this session. She had achieved her goal of separating from her mother while maintaining a healthier relationship with her.

Reflection

This vignette illustrates the use of multiple music therapy approaches, plus art, in the therapy process. Although by this time in our work together Elinor had developed an understanding of the impact on her own psychological and emotional development of her mother's illness and was beginning to release her guilt about wanting to live her own life, she had never allowed herself to fully feel or express the underlying deeply repressed anger and hurt. The BMGIM session had symbolized her sense of abandonment and ultimately uncovered her hurt and anger. The drumming allowed her to express these feelings without words and finally release the painful feelings she had been warding off. After the release, she was supported, grounded, and comforted by music in the Music Imagery experience through imagery in her drawing. This catharsis was supported by the preparation and cognitive understanding she had developed through the 2 years of BMGIM work that preceded these two sessions. It was necessary for her to embody her cognitive learning, which she accomplished through the cathartic release of her drumming.

Fourth Clinical Vignette

Betty

Music therapy approach: Improvisation

Psychodynamic concepts: Making the unconscious conscious
Accessing, "working through," and resolving an issue through music and verbal experiences
Music receives the split-off parts of self and other
Music holds and expresses transference and countertransference responses

In the following clinical vignette. Benedikte Scheiby writes about how she used her musical countertransference "that countertransference that arises during the music experience itself" to understand her 30-year-old female client, an aspiring singer.

[She] wanted to work on her anxiety and nervousness that surfaced every time she was going to perform. The anxiety made it impossible for her to continue singing a song, and she would stop. Betty defined her primary goals as coping with her anxiety, allowing herself to accept her own range of emotions and to avoid being cut off from them, stopping smoking, and becoming more economically independent from her mother. The theme for the improvisation was: "Singing and playing my anxiety."

. . . Betty starts playing tremolos on the piano. I am saying: "I will see if I can try to be there with you when you need it." I accompany her on the metallophone and as soon as I enter the music Betty's music becomes very loud on the piano and vocally in a gradually increasing volume. I get the feeling of being silenced on my metallophone. Betty begins vocalizing with a forced vocal quality. She plays loud clusters at the piano. I reflect Betty's expression vocally, which sounds like a child crying. Another vocal and instrumental outburst from her and she is sighing loudly. Then she starts a fast jazzy melody . . . in the upper register of the piano. It repeats itself. It has a staccato quality just like the beginning playing on the piano. This sounds like a sudden shift to me and I get somewhat puzzled. I listen. I start accompanying on a cymbal. When I play it feels like I am just an appendix underlining the soloist—the pianist.

Betty sings, "I cannot let words out, I cannot let words out"; music therapjst [sic] sings: "I am wondering why, I am wondering why." She is repeating the same words. Music therapist sings: "I am empty for words, I am empty for words, but this is how I feel." Betty starts scatting; I think I hear the word "shut down" in her vocalizing.

Betty singing: "Death is coming" and moves gradually down in the bottom of the register of the piano. I am repeating the sentence with a deep voice following the dynamic of her piano playing.

With no transition, Betty goes over to the big gong and uses it as a background and starts singing very loudly: "Take me over sweet sound. I am loosing [sic] my voice—take me away—I am losing my voice—take me over." The voice becomes playful and she sings: "I guess there is nothing to be afraid of" and slowly scats out of the improvisation.

After a short break she comes over to me and says, "It is interesting, I just realized—I have a lot of instruments at home—it is important that somebody is with me—otherwise I would be doing this at home, wouldn't I?" (Scheiby, 2005, p. 12; used with permission)

Reflection

Scheiby noted several countertransference reactions during the improvisation. Among them were feeling like a young child forced to be silenced by the loud dynamic of the client, and feeling a slight sense of fear move through her body when the client played very loud clusters on the piano. It made her wonder if the client had been forced to be quiet in close relationships at an early age. And she realized there was a clear dynamic with someone taking up a lot of space and the other having very little space. That made her think that that could be a reflection of the relationship between the mother and the child. She also wondered if her somatically experienced fear might be connected to the anxiety that the client experiences when she sings, and she wondered if this fear might have been present in the client every time she was exposed to verbal or physical abuse. These impressions were confirmed by the client.

> In the verbal processing after the improvisation, Betty shared that during the improvisation she had a rush of a pounding headache, which reminded her of the fact that her father often hit her in her head when she was a young child to punish her when "she was crazy"—he "silenced" her. She was also reminded of a punishing situation where she was starting to walk as a young toddler and wanted to touch some things. Her mother had said: "Don't touch that—I will hit you," which eventually happened when the client would touch things. It also reminded her of the physical and sexual abuse that she had been exposed to by a family member. She had often been told that she was a "brat" and a "show off." Betty also said: "I want autonomy and to be separated from my past." And a little later, while she is crying: "Why did they do that to me? I am so angry! My mother came to my mind—I hate her—I want separation." (Scheiby, 2005, p. 13)

Scheiby noted that if the client had not been able to verbalize at this point, she might have asked open-ended questions related to her countertransference impressions. But that was not necessary in this case because the client was able to talk about her experience with great insight. It might also be noted that the client experienced a transference response when Scheiby entered the music, which was manifest in the client's loud playing. This transference elicited Scheiby's countertransference of being silenced. This is a very good illustration of how the client's transference can play a part in the therapist's countertransference. It is clear in this vignette how both transference and countertransference can be used to gain insight into the client's issues for both therapist and client. The intersubjective matrix is a rich source of material that can move the client's process forward. Also illustrated here is how improvisational music can illuminate the client's inner process, bringing to consciousness important early life events that impact present day functioning. In addition, this is an example of the improvisational approach where the therapist fully participates with the client in the improvisational experience.

Case Study

Nancy

Music therapy approach:	Client-selected music listening Lyric analysis
Psychodynamic concepts:	Making the unconscious conscious Accessing, "working through," and resolving issues through music and verbal experiences Resistance and intersubjective collusion Transference and countertransference Music as a container and holding environment Music as a transitional object

Nancy was a 38-year-old single, white physician who came to me with full posttraumatic stress symptoms. She was having nightmares, crying frequently and had difficulty concentrating. She couldn't understand why she was reacting this way, because she herself had not experienced trauma. However, her sister's stepchildren, their mother, stepfather, and another family of four, friends of the family, had all died tragically in an auto accident 2 weeks prior to our meeting. She had traveled to where her sister lived to help out and provide support. Nancy presented as an intelligent, rather inarticulate, soft-spoken woman. She was petite, with blond curly hair, and sat on the couch in my office with her feet curled up under her. She offered details of the accident and her family's response quite readily. However, she was closed down emotionally, unable to access feelings, other than demonstrating a mild sadness and talking about anger toward her mother, but the anger was not evident. I felt a large distance between us.

Nancy was unable to express herself in improvisational music, in imagery, or with art. She was unable to image, either with music or through drawings. Her artistic attempts were very sparse and lacked color. Her attempts at improvisational music were meager as well. In addition, she was unable to attribute any meaning to any of her expressions. Further, she said she never remembered her dreams. It seemed that all possible avenues to her inner world were blocked. In contrast, she was very eager to work on this problem and was interested in music therapy because she sang and played the guitar for relaxation. However, she was so shut down that she could not really engage with any of the experiential activities that were offered to her.

Nancy is the third of four children, one of whom is the developmentally disabled twin of a brother who died at age 16 of a chronic illness. Her sister, 2 years younger, who had just lost her stepchildren in the accident, lives on the East Coast, as does her mother and father who are divorced and living with second spouses. Nancy described her mother as uncaring and said her anger with her was that she acted like she was so concerned during the crisis, and Nancy felt it was all an act.

Her older brother, with whom she was very close, died rather suddenly during a brief hospitalization after an exacerbation of his illness. Nancy, who was 14 years old at the time, stated that her mother blamed her because Nancy had had an argument with him the day before he went to the hospital. She was devasted by her brother's death and said her family didn't seem to know or care how she felt. She was sent to camp for a month a few weeks after her brother's death so that her mother could take a vacation to deal with the loss of her son. Nancy felt completely abandoned. All of this was stated in a matter-of-fact way, without evidence of emotion connected with her story. It became clear that she had not fully grieved her brother's loss and the current deaths had triggered the feelings around the loss of her brother, including anger with her mother about her own abandonment in her time of need.

Nancy's inability to express herself adequately in any arts medium or to find any meaning in what she did produce could be understood as resistance to treatment, arising because something in her psyche must be kept from awareness. However, current intersubjective and relational theories have reframed resistance to mean that it is interpersonal, arising from a collusion between patient and therapist to ensure that nothing new or threatening will occur. I needed to pay attention to my countertransference responses to Nancy's presentation. Resistant behavior in therapy is also seen as an unconscious effort of the patient to communicate with the therapist by evoking in the therapist what she cannot bear alone (Wallin, 1998).

In this context, I was aware of feeling how painful it must have been for Nancy to lose her brother who had been her only ally in her family, and how lonely and abandoned she must have felt at the tender age of 14, with no one to help her manage her overwhelming loss. The only way she could deal with all this was to repress those feelings. Now, in the wake of this tragic accident, all of those feelings had come rushing back, and again, she had to numb herself, the feelings manifest in the PTSD symptoms. I had an image of her as a small, lost child. Further, I also realized that I felt a sense of panic and helplessness that this therapy seemed to be going nowhere. Through this reflection, I understood how I might be colluding with Nancy to protect her (and perhaps myself as well) from these feelings. I also understood her sense of helplessness and desperation. This realization ended the collusion. I decided to ask her to bring in music that expressed significant moments in her life.

The first tape she brought in was one of herself singing and accompanying herself on the guitar. It was a song called "Flyin' Shoes." Her voice was very childlike and plaintive. The lyrics were about being tired of the "same old blues, same old song," and expressed the wish to go far away on "Flyin' Shoes." She said when she taped the song, she felt the sadness and loneliness, but did not feel it as we listened to her recording. I interpreted for her that those feelings probably represented what she had felt as a child, and in particular around her brother's death. She said maybe, but maybe she was just making it up. She had internalized her mother's attitude toward her and did not trust her own internal experience.

At the next session she brought in an a cappella song sung by three Congolese women who were mourning the drowning of a child. She related this directly to her brother's death and said the music sounded like she felt at that time. The women's voices are wailing in very beautiful mournful tones. We sat in silence and listened to it two or three times. Again, she said she could not really feel the feelings during the session, but had felt them at home when she made the selection. I also wondered if the selection of African singers was an expression of an unconscious wish to please me or relate to me as an African American woman, an attempt to bridge some of the distance between us, and perhaps the beginning of a positive transference with me. I did not make this interpretation to her because it was more important to stay with the meaning of the song for her, a conscious expression of mourning her brother.

Nancy also brought in another song that she related to her brother's death, called "Barbed Wire." This was a lively country western song with an upbeat tempo, sung by a male singer with guitar accompaniment. The lyrics, however, were about how barbed wire "locks me out and locks you in. It hurts so deep inside." Her initial associations to this were about feeling withdrawn from the family. We were both aware of how easily one could get hurt trying to go through barbed wire, making any attempt on her part to bridge the gap between her and her mother a dangerous undertaking. A few weeks later she realized that the barbed wire was also how she perceived her mother as locking her out when her brother died. She was in touch with the line that said, "People keep you out at any cost, never knowing how much it hurts." It's very likely that the upbeat nature of this music helped Nancy to connect with the painful lyrics. The music itself bound her anxiety sufficiently to allow her to approach the repressed feelings. In other words, the music itself may have acted as a transitional object helping her tolerate the painful feelings contained in the lyrics.

An interesting aspect of this therapy was that Nancy had so much difficulty expressing herself in the therapy room. This was probably at least partially transference, because her mother was a psychologist and psychotherapist, and she clearly did not trust her mother. It seemed that this transference inhibited her ability to become more vulnerable with me. However, she was able to establish sufficient trust with the music, and through it with me, to have a positive therapeutic experience.

Through these songs, Nancy was able to bring her repressed feelings to consciousness and use the music to tolerate them. Her nightmares and frequent tearfulness subsided and she regained her ability to concentrate. Although she realized she still had work to do related to her mother, she was able to return to work and was ready to stop therapy for now. She wanted to turn her energy to planning her upcoming wedding. She had accomplished her goal of relieving the symptoms that brought her into therapy.

Reflection

This case demonstrates how client-selected music can unlock repressed feelings and bring relief from debilitating symptoms. Although Nancy was not able to be emotionally demonstrative in my presence, the music obviously touched her deeply and allowed her to grieve her brother and begin to heal an old wound. It also demonstrates the effectiveness of the therapist exploring the intersubjective matrix and recognizing how through her countertransference, she can collude with the client's anxieties and fears to ward off the client's repressed feelings. When I recognized my feelings as representative of what she was probably feeling and understood that I was protecting her (and myself) by not finding a way into her grief, the therapeutic process moved ahead and Nancy worked through a good deal of the trauma that led to the posttraumatic stress symptoms. This case also illustrates how the client's transference can interfere with the therapeutic alliance and how the therapist has to be cognizant of these effects and act to mitigate them when the client is unable to work with the transference directly.

Conclusions

We have arrived at a stage in the development of our field in which many authors are expounding on all aspects of psychodynamic music therapy. Despite the apparent differences, there are some fundamental concepts that are shared by most psychodynamic music therapists. Psychodynamic music therapy, simply stated, is based on the concept that events in the past have an impact on the present and that unconscious material drives current behavior. The goal of therapy is to uncover and work through the past and unconscious elements that interfere with current functioning. Although the degree to which the musical experience versus the verbal exchange is viewed as being an agent of change may vary among psychodynamic music therapists, most would consider the triadic relationships among the client, the music, and the therapist (Summer, 1998) to be essential ingredients of the therapeutic process.

Psychodynamic music therapy focuses on questions of meaning. The level of inquiry in which we must engage to arrive at answers forces us to stretch our limits, intellectually and clinically. Whereas Streeter (1999) begins the construction of a theory of "musical transference" (p. 85), Odell (1988) looks at the therapist's way of responding musically to the patient as a form of interpretation. Our need to move from the verbal to the musical level and back involves us in a complex process. As we, psychodynamic music therapists, make our way in the professional community and as we try to find our place within the community of mental health professionals, we must define ourselves as therapists with the advanced training and in-depth skills required to allow us to focus on depth therapy.

Psychodynamic music therapists must have advanced musical skills and, specifically, improvisational skills. Musical freedom is required to respond to patients' musical productions within an improvisational music therapy context. In addition, to use receptive music therapy effectively, psychodynamic music therapists must have knowledge of a wide range of musical genres and an understanding of how the various musical elements impact the individual emotionally, psychologically, physically, and spiritually. Psychotherapeutic skills are mandatory for this work. Training must occur at an advanced academic level. Personal experience in psychotherapy or in psychodynamic music therapy, although not a requirement in all settings, is highly desirable. For if, as Freud (1915/2001) said, "the Ucs. [unconscious] of one human being can react upon that of another, without passing through the Cs. [conscious]" (p. 194), then we, as therapists, have the responsibility of becoming aware of our own unconscious.

References

Ahonen-Eerikainen,H. (2004) Musically elicited images as unique clinical data during the process of group analysis with traumatised adults. *British Journal of Music Therapy, 18*, 24–29.

Ahonen-Eerikainen,H. (2007). *Group analytic music therapy*. Gilsum, NH: Barcelona.

Aigen, K. (1995). An aesthetic foundation of clinical theory: An underlying basis of Creative Music Therapy. In C. Kenny (Ed.), *Listening, playing, creating: Essays on the power of sound* (pp. 233–257). Albany, NY: SUNY.

Alvin, J. (1975). *Music therapy*. London: Hutchinson.

Austin, D. (1991). The musical mirror: Music therapy for the narcissistically injured. In K. Bruscia (Ed.), *Case studies in music therapy* (pp. 291–307). Gilsum, NH: Barcelona.

Austin, D. (1996). The role of improvised music in psychodynamic music therapy with adults. *Music Therapy, 14*(1), pp. 29–43.

Austin, D. (1999). Vocal improvisation in analytically oriented music therapy with adults. In T. Wigram & J. De Backer (Eds.), *Clinical applications of music therapy in psychiatry* (pp. 141–157). London: Jessica Kingsley.

Austin, D., & Dvorkin, J. (1998). Resistance in individual music therapy. In K. Bruscia (Ed.), *The dynamics of music psychotherapy* (pp. 121–135). Gilsum, NH: Barcelona.

Bonny, H. L. (2002). Guided Imagery and Music (GIM): Mirror of consciousness. In H. Bonny (L. Summer, Ed.), *Music and consciousness: The evolution of Guided Imagery and Music* (pp. 93–102). Gilsum, NH: Barcelona.

Bruscia, K. (1998a). *Defining music therapy* (2nd ed.). Gilsum, NH: Barcelona.

Bruscia, K. (Ed.). (1998b). *The dynamics of music psychotherapy*. Gilsum, NH: Barcelona.

Bruscia, K. (1998c). An introduction to music psychotherapy. In K. Bruscia (Ed.), *The dynamics of music psychotherapy* (pp. 1–15). Gilsum, NH: Barcelona.

Darnley-Smith, R., & Patey, H. M. (2003). *Music therapy*. London: Sage.

Detrick, D., & Detrick, S. (Eds.). (1989). *Self psychology: Comparisons and contrasts.* Hillsdale, NJ: The Analytic Press.

Diaz de Chumaceiro, C. (1998). Unconsciously induced song recall. In K. Bruscia (Ed.), *The dynamics of music psychotherapy* (pp. 335–363). Gilsum, NH: Barcelona.

Dillard, L.M. (2006). Musical countertransference experiences of music therapists: A phenomenological study. *The Arts in Psychotherapy, 33*, 208–217.

Dvorkin, J., & Erlund, M. (2003). The girl who barked: Object Relations music psychotherapy with an eleven-year-old autistic female. In S. Hadley (Ed.), *Psychodynamic music therapy: Case studies* (pp. 183–203). Gilsum, NH: Barcelona.

Erkkilä, J. (2004). From signs to symbols, from symbols to words: About the relationship between music and language, music therapy and psychotherapy. *Voices: A World Forum for Music Therapy, 4*(2). Retrieved July 22, 2008, from http://www.voices.no/main issues/mi40003000150.html

Eschen, J. Th. (Ed.). (2002). *Analytical music therapy.* London: Jessica Kingsley.

Eyre, L. (2007). Changes in images, life events and music in Analytical Music Therapy: A reconstruction of Mary Priestley's case study of "Curtis" In A. Meadows (Ed.), *Qualitative inquiries in music therapy: A monograph series* (Vol. 3, pp. 1–30). Gilsum, NH: Barcelona.

Freud, S. (1915/2001). *The unconscious. The standard edition of the complete psychological works of Sigmund Freud* (Vol. 14, pp. 159–215). London: Hogarth Press.

Freud, S. (1926/2001). *The question of lay analysis. The standard edition of the complete psychological works of Sigmund Freud* (Vol. 20, pp. 177–250). London: Hogarth Press.

Goldberg, F. (2000). I am the creator and the created: A woman's journey from loss to wholeness. *Beiträge zur Musiktherapie, 10,* 47–58.

Hadley, S. (2003). *Psychodynamic music therapy: Case studies.* Gilsum, NH: Barcelona.

Heimann, P. (1950). On counter-transference. *International Journal of Psychoanalysis, 31,* 81–84.

Inada, M. (2007). From performer to container: A psychiatric group with a musically accomplished client. *British Journal of Music Therapy, 21,* 53–57.

Isenberg-Grzeda, C. (1989). Therapist self-disclosure in music therapy practice. *Proceedings of the Sixteenth Annual Conference of the Canadian Association for Music Therapy,* Ottawa, pp. 49–54.

Isenberg-Grzeda, C. (1998). Transference structures in Guided Imagery and Music. In K. Bruscia (Ed.), *The dynamics of music psychotherapy* (pp. 461–479). Gilsum, NH: Barcelona.

Jahn-Langenberg, M. (2003). Harmony and dissonance in conflict: Psychoanalytically informed music therapy with a psychosomatic patient. In S. Hadley (Ed.), *Psychodynamic music therapy: Case studies* (pp. 357–373). Gilsum, NH: Barcelona.

Kenny, C. (1989). *The field of play: A guide for the theory and practice of music therapy.* Atascadero, CA: Ridgeview.

Lecourt, E. (1993). *Analyse de groupe et musicothérapie.* Paris: ESF.

Lecourt, E. (1994). *L'expérience musicale résonances psychanalytiques.* Paris: Editions L'Harmattan.

Lecourt, E. (2004). The psychic functions of music. *Nordic Journal of Music Therapy, 13,* 154–160.

Lipson, C. T. (2006). The meanings and functions of tunes that come into one's head. *Psychoanalytic Quarterly, 75,* 859–878.

Marom, M. (2008). "Patient declined": Contemplating the psychodynamics of hospice music therapy. *Music Therapy Perspectives, 26*, 13–22.

McKinney, C. (1993). The case of Therese: Multidimensional growth through Guided Imagery and Music. *Journal of the Association for Music and Imagery, 2*, 99–109.

Metzner, S. (2004). Some thoughts on receptive music therapy from a psychoanalytic viewpoint. *Nordic Journal of Music Therapy, 13,* 143–150.

Moore, B., & Fine, B. (Eds.). (1990). *Psychoanalytic terms and concepts.* New Haven, CT: Yale University Press.

Nolan, P. (1994). The therapeutic response in improvisational music therapy: What goes on inside? *Music Therapy Perspectives, 12*, 84–91.

Nolan, P. (2003). Through music to therapeutic attachment: Psychodynamic music therapy with a musician with dysthymic disorder. In S. Hadley (Ed.), *Psychodynamic music therapy: Case studies* (pp. 319–338). Gilsum, NH: Barcelona.

Odell, H. (1988). A music therapy approach in mental health. *Psychology of Music, 16*(1), 52–62.

Pavlicevic, M. (1997). *Music therapy in context.* London: Jessica Kingsley.

Pavlicevic, M. (1999). *Music therapy: Intimate notes.* London: Jessica Kingsley.

Priestley, M. (1975). *Music therapy in action.* London: Constable.

Priestley, M. (1994). *Essays on Analytical Music Therapy.* Phoenixville, PA: Barcelona.

Priestley, M., & Eschen, J. Th. (2002). Analytical Music Therapy—Origin and development. In J. Th. Eschen (Ed.), *Analytical Music Therapy* (pp. 11–16). London: Jessica Kingsley.

Robarts, J. (2003). The healing function of improvised songs in music therapy with a child survivor of early trauma and sexual abuse. In S. Hadley (Ed.), *Psychodynamic music therapy: Case studies* (pp. 141–182). Gilsum, NH: Barcelona.

Rusbridger, R. (2008). The internal world of Don Giovanni. *The International Journal of Psychoanalysis, 89*, 181–194.

Ruud, E. (1980). *Music therapy and its relationship to current treatment theories.* St. Louis, MO: Magnamusic-Baton.

Salmon, D. (2008). Bridging music and psychoanalytic therapy. *Voices: A World Forum for Music Therapy.* Retrieved July 19, 2008, from http://www.voices.no/mainissues/mi40008000260.php

Scheiby, B. (2005). An intersubjective approach to music therapy: Identification and processing of musical countertransference in a music psychotherapeutic context. *Music Therapy Perspectives, 23*(1), 8–17.

Schmidt-Peters, J. (2000). *Music therapy: An introduction* (2nd ed.). Springfield: Charles C. Thomas.

Schneider, E. H., Unkefer, R., & Gaston, E. T. (1968). Introduction. In E. T. Gaston (Ed.), *Music in therapy* (pp. 1–4). New York: Macmillan.

Silverman, M. J. (2007). Evaluating current trends in psychiatric music therapy: A descriptive analysis. *Journal of Music Therapy, 44*, 388–414.

Stein, A. (2004). Music, mourning, and consolation. *Journal of the American Psychoanalytic Association, 52*, 783–811.

Stolorow, R., Brandshaft, B., & Atwood, G. (1987). *Psychoanalytic treatment: An intersubjective approach.* Hillsdale, NJ: The Analytic Press.

Streeter, E. (1999). Definition and use of the musical transference relationship. In T. Wigram & J. De Backer (Eds.), *Clinical applications of music therapy in psychiatry* (pp. 84–101). London: Jessica Kingsley.

Summer, L. (1998). The pure music transference in Guided Imagery and Music. In K. Bruscia (Ed.), *The dynamics of music psychotherapy* (pp. 431–459). Gilsum, NH: Barcelona.

Turry, A. (1998). Transference and countertransference in Nordoff-Robbins music therapy. In K. Bruscia (Ed.), *The dynamics of music psychotherapy* (pp. 161–212). Gilsum, NH: Barcelona.

Tyson, F. (1965). Therapeutic elements in out-patient music therapy. *The Psychoanalytic Quarterly*, 315–327.

Tyson, F. (1981). *Psychiatric music therapy.* New York: Creative Arts Rehabilitation Center.

Wallin, D. (1998). *Intersubjectivity and relational theory: How the new paradigm transforms the way we work.* Mill Valley, CA: Psychotherapy Tape Works, Marin Psychotherapy Institute.

Wärja, M. (1994). Sounds of music through the spiraling path of individuation: A Jungian approach to music psychotherapy. *Music Therapy Perspectives, 12,* 75–83.

Wheeler, B. (1981). The relationship between music therapy and theories of psychotherapy. *Music Therapy, 1*(1), 9–16.

Wheeler, B. (1983). A psychotherapeutic classification of music therapy practices: A continuum of procedures. *Music Therapy Perspectives, 1*(2), 8–12.

Wheeler, B. (1987). Levels of therapy: The classification of music therapy goals. *Music Therapy, 6*(2), 39–49.

Wigram, T., & De Backer, J. (1999). *Clinical applications of music therapy in psychiatry.* London: Jessica Kingsley.

Wigram, T., Pedersen, I. N., & Bonde, L. O. (2002). *A comprehensive guide to music therapy.* London: Jessica Kingsley.

Winnicott, D. W. (1971). *Playing and reality.* New York: Penguin Books.

Wolberg, L. R. (1977). *The technique of psychotherapy* (3rd ed.). New York: Grune & Stratton.

Wolf, E. (1988). *Treating the self.* New York: The Guilford Press.

Research Resources

Aldridge, D. (1996). *Music therapy research and practice in medicine.* London: Jessica Kingsley. Briefly reviews the published research in music therapy in the areas of psychiatry and psychotherapy.

Aldridge, D. (1996). *Music therapy info CD-Rom I.* Witten/Herdecke: Universitat Witten/Herdecke.

Aldridge, D. (1998). *Music therapy info CD-Rom II.* Witten/Herdecke: Universitat Witten/ Herdecke.

Aldridge, D. (2001). *Music therapy info CD-Rom III.* Witten/Herdecke: Universitat Witten/ Herdecke.

Aldridge, D., & Fachner, J. (2002). *Music therapy world info CD-Rom IV.* Witten/Herdecke: Universitat Witten/Herdecke.

Wigram, T., Pedersen, I. N., & Bonde, L. O. (2002). Music therapy research and clinical assessment. In T. Wigram & F. M. Hughes (Eds.), *A comprehensive guide to music therapy* (pp. 221–266). London: Jessica Kingsley.

Recommended Additional Readings

Brenner, C. (1973). *An elementary textbook of psychoanalysis* (Rev. ed.). Garden City, NY: Anchor Press.

Bruscia, K., & Grocke, D. (Eds.). (2002). *Guided Imagery and Music: The Bonny Method and beyond.* Gilsum, NH: Barcelona.

Freud, S. (1900/2001). *The interpretation of dreams. The standard edition of the complete psychological works of Sigmund Freud* (Vols. 4 & 5). London: Hogarth Press.

Goldberg, F. (1995). The Bonny Method of Guided Imagery and Music. In T. Wigram, B. Saperston, & R. West (Eds.), *The art and science of music therapy: A handbook* (pp. 112–128). Switzerland: Hardwood Academic.

Greenberg, J. R., & Mitchell, S. A. (1983). *Object relations in psychoanalytic theory.* Cambridge, MA: Harvard University Press.

Jung, C. J. (Ed.). (1964). *Man and his symbols.* New York: Dell.

Jung, C. J. (1972). *Two essays on analytical psychology* (2nd ed.; R. F. C. Hull, Trans.). Princeton, NJ: Princeton University Press.

Kast, V. (1992). *The dynamics of symbols.* New York: Fromm International.

Kohut, H. (1984). *How does analysis cure?* Chicago: The University of Chicago Press.

Natterson, J., & Friedman, R. (1995). *A primer of clinical intersubjectivity.* Northvale, NJ: Jason Aronson.

Pine, F. (1990). *Drive, ego, object and self.* New York: Basic Books.

Ruitenbeek, H. M. (Ed.). (1973). *The first Freudians.* New York: Jason Aronson.

Stolorow, R., Atwood, G., & Brandshaft, B. (Eds.). (1994). *The intersubjective experience.* Northvale, NJ: Jason Aronson.

Winnicott, D. W. (1971). *Collected papers: Through pediatrics to psycho-analysis.* London: Tavistock.

Wollheim, R. (1971). *Freud.* Glasgow, Scotland: Fontana/Collins.

Chapter 8

Behavioral Approach to Music Therapy

Jane Standley
Christopher M. Johnson
Sheri L. Robb
Mike D. Brownell
Shin-Hee Kim

Introduction

Psychotherapy and the field of psychology have been dominated through most of the last 50 years by a science known as behaviorism. Over four centuries ago, a new trend in Western thought emerged that led to the rise of behaviorism and was characterized by (a) movement toward empirical testing of hypotheses and away from reliance on authority, (b) movement toward physicalism and away from mental events, and (c) movement toward belief in science and away from mysticism. By the end of the 19th century, this view toward positivism dominated philosophical thinking. Early behaviorism was an extension of positivism and rejected any hypothesis that did not lead to physically quantifiable and measurable behavior (Baars, 1986).

Behaviorism resulted in a strong movement to create a psychology that would allow for objective study of the human mind and behavior. Rather than focusing on analysis of consciousness, these new psychologists developed empirical theories by studying human behavior via the methods of the physical sciences: established research methods, formal experimental designs, and statistical analyses of results (Baars, 1986; Wilson, 2000).

Behaviorism comprises the philosophical and theoretical foundations of this science, while applied behavior analysis is the basic research component. B. F. Skinner (1904–1990), in addition to being the recognized founder of the experimental analysis of behavior, wrote extensively on its philosophy. Though a common view is that behaviorism rejects all events that cannot be operationally defined by objective assessment, this view is naïve and simply incorrect. The philosophy of behaviorism clearly acknowledges the importance of private events. Skinner himself referred to events taking place "inside the skin." A behaviorist would consider it a mistake to rule out inaccessible, internal events that influence human behavior. Rather, this approach seeks to assign a constructed model of cognitive process as the explanation for that which can be observed.

Out of behaviorism emerged behavior therapy. During the late 1950s, behavior therapy began using a systematic, research-based approach to the assessment and treatment of psychological disorders (Eifert & Plaud, 1998; Masters, Burish, Hollon, & Rimm, 1987). Initially, this new treatment approach was defined as the application of modern learning theory (the principles of operant and classical conditioning) to the treatment of clinical problems (Wilson, 2000). As all science evolves across time, behavior therapy has undergone major changes and currently includes cognitive-behavioral approaches for resolving psychological problems. Both are widely accepted and highly effective psychotherapies widely utilized by music therapists in educational, medical, and psychiatric settings. A recent survey by Silverman (2007b) found that 83.1% of music therapists in psychiatric settings reported using behavioral methodologies.

Primary Approaches to Contemporary Behavior Therapy

There are three distinct approaches to contemporary behavior therapy. Applied behavior analysis today still relies on the principles of operant conditioning set forth by B. F. Skinner, which maintains that behavior is a function of its consequences; therefore, therapeutic interventions emphasize changing the relationship between overt behaviors and their consequences (Skinner, 1948, 1953). Techniques identified with applied behavior analysis include reinforcement, punishment, extinction, contingencies, token economies, and stimulus control. A second approach expands these techniques and encompasses a mediational stimulus-response model that applies the principles of classical conditioning derived from the work of Ivan Pavlov, E. R. Guthrie, Clark Hull, and Joseph Wolpe, with acknowledgment of intervening or mediational variables (Wheeler, 1981; Wilson, 2000). Since covert or cognitive processes are believed to follow the same laws of learning that govern overt behaviors, it is assumed that mediational variables are subject to modification. Techniques related to the mediational stimulus-response model include flooding, systematic desensitization, and imagery (Wheeler, 1981; Wilson, 2000).

As theoretical and research bases of behavior therapy began to expand toward the end of the 1960s, behavior therapists began to explore therapeutic strategies from social, personality, and developmental psychology. During this time, Bandura's social learning theory emerged. Social learning theory asserts that man is neither internally impelled nor a passive responder to the environment, but a choosing individual engaging in reciprocal interaction with his or her environment (Bandura, 1969). Primary characteristics of social learning theory include vicarious learning (modeling), symbolic processes, and self-regulation. Recognition of self-regulatory processes led to newer forms of therapy, known as social-cognitive therapy. This therapy views behavior as dependent on three separate but interacting regulatory processes that include (a) external stimulus events, (b) external reinforcement, and (c) cognitive mediational processes. How an individual perceives and interprets events that occur within the environment, therefore, determines behavior. The social-cognitive therapeutic approach emphasizes self-directed behavior change (Wilson, 2000).

An increase in the presence of cognitive processes and procedures in behavior therapy in the 1970s was followed by increased attention to the role of affect in therapeutic change during the

1980s and 1990s. In recent years, behavior therapists have begun to take interest in the complex interactions that occur among behavior, cognition, and affect (Thaut, 1989). Arnold Lazarus operationalized this interaction by focusing on the firing order, or triggers, of human responses, i.e., the angry person who immediately attacks (behavior) before thinking (cognition) versus the irritated person who endlessly mulls over a perceived slight (cognition) until it acquires dramatic proportion, then attacks (behavior). Intervention focuses on tracking, then altering the firing order of social, emotional, cognitive, and behavioral responses to interrupt the undesirable series of events (Wilson, 2000).

A Brief History of Behaviorism in Music Therapy

Behaviorism and Music Therapy in the Early Years (1948-1970)

The professions of music therapy and behavior therapy evolved during the same time period. The therapeutic application of behavioral principles was first realized in an article published in the *American Journal of Psychology* by Fuller (1949), reporting the effect of a primary reinforcer on movement of the subject's arm. The formal beginning of applied behavior analysis was the publication of a paper by Ayllon and Michael (1959), "The Psychiatric Nurse as a Behavioral Engineer" (Cooper, Heron, & Heward, 1987). There were three other landmark publications in the 1960s. The first two were a pair of books by Ullman and Krasner that reported studies in one book (Ullman & Krasner, 1965) using a set of techniques outlined by the other text (Krasner & Ullman, 1965). A further important event during this period was the 1968 publication of the *Journal of Applied Behavior Analysis* that was and continues to be the premier journal in the area of behavioral psychology.

During the time behaviorism was in its infancy, music therapy began as a formal area of study. Following World War II, there was an increased demand for music therapy services for persons who served in the military. This demand resulted in the emergence of degree programs in higher education during the 1940s and the formation of a national professional organization, The National Association for Music Therapy, in 1950 (Clair, 1996; Davis, Gfeller, & Thaut, 2008).

A strong behavioral presence is found in the philosophical viewpoints and writings of professionals in music therapy during the 1960s and 1970s. Gaston (1968), a prominent early leader in music therapy, called for the scientific exploration of therapeutic music interventions using a behavioral approach. Gaston regarded music as a form of human behavior and felt that scientific investigation of the "feelingful aspects" of life was imperative. Esther Goetz Gilliland (1962) argued that human response to musical stimuli is a conditioned response, clearly reflecting the principles of classical conditioning. Sears (1968) provided a framework for the objective classification of behavior and outlined continua of behavior to facilitate a better theoretical understanding of the function of music in therapy.

The *Journal of Music Therapy* (*JMT*), established in 1964, was dedicated to the research efforts of music therapists. Two early publications in the *JMT* introduced a behavioral approach to music therapy and the application of behavioral research techniques (Madsen & Madsen, 1968; Steele, 1977). Gfeller's (1987) review of *JMT* literature between 1964 and 1984 provides additional evidence of strong ties between behaviorism and music therapy. Gfeller found that early volumes of the *JMT* referred primarily to psychoanalytic principles. The frequency of these references to psychoanalysis, however, declined from 1964 to 1979, and a sudden increase in behavioral approaches was evident. Gfeller concluded that behavioral and psychoanalytic approaches remained the dominant theoretical orientations of the profession during these early years.

Behaviorism and Music Therapy in the Latter Years (1980-present)

An examination of contemporary literature serves to illustrate the continued prominence of behaviorism in music therapy practice and reveals the emergence of both cognitive and affective components. In the 1970s, many music therapy publications described interventions based on the principles of operant and classical conditioning (Dorow, 1975; Madsen & Madsen, 1968; McCarty, McElfresh, Rice, & Wilson, 1978). Acceptance of behavioral music therapy as a primary psychotherapy soon followed (Hanser, 1983; Scovel, 1990; Wheeler, 1981).

Recent movement toward cognitive-behavioral approaches in music therapy stayed abreast of changes in behavior therapy. First to appear in the music therapy literature was Rational Emotive Therapy (RET) developed by Albert Ellis (Bryant, 1987; Maultsby, 1977). In 1987, Bryant described a cognitive approach to music interventions based on the principles of RET. According to Bryant, a person's relationship to music provides a manifestation of his or her values, attitudes, and beliefs, both rational and irrational. The therapist, therefore, can use music to assist clients in detection, clarification, examination, debate, and refutation of distorted or irrational beliefs. Ellis himself advocates the use of humorous music to trigger cognitive change (Ellis, 1987), and the Rational-Emotive Institute distributes a tape of him singing his favorite selections (Ellis, 2003).

Thaut (1989) described the role of affect modification in behavioral learning and change, as well as the connection between affect, cognition, and behavior. In this approach, the music therapist uses the affective and motivational qualities in music perception to modify mood. Due to the direct link between emotions and learning, Thaut advocated that traditional cognitive and behavioral therapies would be complemented by methods that evoke emotions and influence mood states.

Selm (1991) presented a cognitive-behavioral treatment model for chronic pain that marked the emergence of self-regulation techniques in the practice of music therapy. The author advocated the use of a multidimensional approach wherein the music therapist reinforces the acquisition of new information, challenges old beliefs and teaches the client to practice new behaviors, promotes nonverbal expression of emotional states, and promotes the acquisition of self-regulation skills. Desensitization to undesirable physical and emotional responses through progressive relaxation and self-regulation techniques such as biofeedback are also prevalent in the music therapy literature (Davis, 1992; Hanser, 1990; Mandel, 1996; McCarthy, 1992; Rider, Floyd, & Kirkpatrick, 1985; Robb, Nichols, Rutan, Bishop, & Parker, 1995; Scartelli, 1984).

There has been dynamic growth in behavioral music therapy and development of diverse techniques over the past 50 years. It is now a major psychotherapy practiced worldwide and characterized by a unique, research-based methodology. In an invited address as a leader of a "founding model" of music therapy presented to the General Assembly of the 9th World Congress of Music Therapy (1999), Clifford Madsen provided this overview:

The theoretical underpinnings of this approach are consistent with other scientific approaches and are intentionally parsimonious, yet very far reaching. Music can be used (1) as a cue, (2) as a time and body movement structure, (3) as a focus of attention, and (4) as a reward. While principles are few, effective application of the behavioral model is extremely complex and requires extensive training for effective intervention. Behavioral music therapy requires a solid understanding of the principles of behavior and a refined ability to analyze, criticize, and choose alternatives necessitating extensive creativity in designing procedures. This approach involves the creation, selection, and improvisation of music idiosyncratic to the specific necessities of dealing with shaping the behavior of each individual patient or client. (Madsen, 1999)

The field continues to develop new theories and effective treatment interventions that are documented through the empirical investigation of these diverse aspects of human functioning and behavior.

Behavioral Techniques Used by Music Therapists

It is the goal of this section to review basic behavioral techniques commonly used in music therapy practice. These techniques can be understood only in the context of four important behavioral principles. The first is that the object of behaviorism is to identify, modify, count, or otherwise observe a behavior or behavioral indicator of a cognitive or affective process. Though most people engaging in behavioral practice acknowledge and even embrace the precepts of cognition and affect, the behavioral approach recognizes evidence of those domains through observable means. An example of this is Robb's (2000) use of operationally defined behaviors of hospitalized children to objectively examine their relationship and involvement with their medical environment. Additionally, Ghetti (2002) examined the effects of various music conditions on observable/measurable behavior states of students with profound disabilities.

Once specified behaviors have been targeted, then observation is utilized to document what events are occurring and their magnitude. This process is completed prior to implementing any behavioral program in order to determine whether the program is necessary, and, if so, to later document progress.

The next step in a behavioral program is to introduce contingencies into the environment to influence the client into modifying his or her behavior in a positive direction. These contingencies can range widely depending on the individual. People who assert that rewards should not be overtly given but intrinsically determined sometimes criticize the use of contingencies as bribery. These same individuals often fail to realize that if they were to stop receiving a paycheck, they would probably stop going to work, or that they seldom leave their child's report card unopened in order to allow the child to intrinsically feel good about the work done at school. Of course, therapists want all individuals to reach the point of independent, intrinsic enlightenment. However, if that naturally happened, there would be no need for therapists. Therefore, purposefully selected contingencies must be established for a period of time if a new behavioral pattern is to be established.

The final step in a behavioral therapy program is to evaluate results through continued or post observation of the targeted behavior. When specified criteria are met, including independence, generalization, and self-sustaining maintenance of the new behavior pattern, then therapy can be terminated. Behavioral therapists are concerned that the client's distress, discomfort, or lack of success be alleviated as quickly and effectively as possible, and they frequently select techniques and procedures on this basis. Behavior therapists also work within an accountability paradigm: the behavior selected prior to treatment must be documented through observable means as changing in the desired way in order to be considered successful. There are several differing scientific designs that can clearly identify whether a given contingency or set of contingencies is working with a particular client. These can be found in many good texts on behavioral techniques or applied behavior analysis (Alberto & Troutman, 1995; Bergin & Garfield, 1994; Cooper et al., 1987; Madsen & Madsen, 1998). Applied behavior analysis, also known as single subject research, excels at providing clinicians with a method to directly test the functional relationship between selected techniques and targeted client behavior (Hanser, 1995). The use of behavioral designs continues to increase in the literature and is particularly practical for clinicians as it does not necessitate large numbers of clients or cumbersome statistical models (Gregory, 2002).

The remainder of this chapter briefly summarizes the many operant and cognitive-behavioral techniques used by behavioral therapists. (Thorough definitions can be found in Madsen and Madsen, 1998.) Presentation of operant techniques is subdivided according to those used for teaching new behaviors, those used to strengthen existing behaviors, and those used to weaken existing behaviors. Classic and important research studies that document the benefits of each technique accompany these descriptions rather than being compiled into a single research overview. The extant research literature in behavioral music therapy is too prolific to be fully included in this chapter.

Operant Techniques

Techniques for teaching new behaviors introduce or structure an environmental antecedent event that will encourage an appropriate behavioral response. Occurrences of the new behavior must be accompanied by immediate and reinforcing feedback. These techniques include task analysis, prompts, fading, errorless learning, chaining, shaping, successive approximations, and modeling.

A *task analysis* is the delineation of a selected activity into its component, sequential parts. Standley (1998) demonstrated the benefits of a hierarchical task analysis of neurological tolerance to increasingly complex stimuli with premature infants in the Neonatal Intensive Care Unit. Music maintained pacification while multimodal stimuli were systematically introduced. Results showed faster habituation indicative of increased neurological maturity and earlier hospital discharge. Also, task analysis principles can be applied to an entire program plan or curriculum design as with the comprehensive music therapy objectives outlined by Darrow, Gfeller, Gorsuch, and Thomas (2000) for children who are deaf or hearing impaired.

A *prompt* is the most basic technique for aiding a client to emit a new response and is simply a cue that increases the probability of a desired response. For example, a child learning to label objects is presented with a ball. If no verbal response occurs, the therapist might produce the beginning speech sound desired, *buh* for ball. Music therapists also use music as a cue to elicit an affective response (new mood) or to cue reminiscence of a patient with Alzheimer's disease. Therapists discard prompts when no longer required to stimulate the desired response. *Fading* is the systematic process of withdrawing these cues or prompts so that behavior becomes independent and habitual.

Errorless learning is a procedure to establish accurate client responses as rapidly as possible without the appearance of errors. For instance, a child with developmental delays is learning to eat with a spoon. The child acquires food on the spoon and moves it directly to his or her mouth while a therapist guides the hand through this process. The guided assistance is faded step-by-step as the client repeats the correct behavior. Using this procedure, the child never engages in the endless possibilities of errors such as throwing the spoon, dropping it to finger feed, putting the spoon in the glass rather than the plate, etc.

Rather than the degree of therapist assistance reducing errors, the task itself can be structured without errors. For example, a child with a behavior disorder who is mainstreamed in a music education chorus may be given the goal of entering the room and sitting in his or her designated chair for rehearsal. The task can be structured for errorless learning usually in one session by beginning the task with only the correct chair in its designated place in the room. The other chairs are systematically and quickly returned as the child repeats the correct behavior of entering the room and sitting in the designated one. Of course, the other chairs are returned according to their proximity to the designated chair, those farthest away added first and those closest added last.

Chaining is the process of two or more responses being joined together systematically, one at a time. As each new behavior is added, the entire sequence to that point is repeatedly practiced. Young children might be taught the alphabet sequence using this procedure: teaching one letter, then a second, then the two in sequence, etc. Wolfe and Horn (1993) implemented a variant of chaining, termed *reverse chaining*, to help preschool children remember their phone numbers. The sequence of numbers was presented under a variety of stimulus conditions, then presented again excluding the last digit. If the child was able to recall the last digit, the phone number was presented again, omitting the last two digits and so on until the child was able to recall the entire phone number. The results of this study showed that the reverse chaining procedure, accompanied by familiar music, was most effective in teaching phone number recall. The music condition also required the fewest number of prompts to recall sequential information presented in the chaining procedures.

Madsen and Madsen (1983) define *successive approximation* as "behavioral elements or subsets, each of which more and more closely resembles the specified terminal behavior" (p. 277). *Shaping* is systematically reinforcing each of those behaviors as they more closely approximate the desired objectives. These two techniques are frequently combined with task analysis. When behavioral therapists teach new behaviors to a client, they begin by using the skills that the client already possesses. Each subsequent step of a detailed task analysis becomes a successive approximation toward the final behavior that is being taught. As each of these steps is mastered, the client is reinforced until the goal behavior is reached.

Successive approximation was used by Eisenstein (1976) to associate musical terminology with correct symbols. Through the course of the experiment, cues and prompts were gradually faded as the pool of symbols increased. The target behavior was to accurately associate 15 musical symbols with their corresponding terminology. The author concluded that successive approximation, when coupled with verbal approval and feedback, was effective in improving academic verbal music behaviors.

Shaping and successive approximation are widely used in behavioral counseling. For instance, a client traumatized by rape may have an aversion to sexual contact even with a beloved partner. When the client is ready to overcome this aversion, the partner might be taught to identify successive approximations of sexual contact and to respond accordingly. The client is never forced into aversive behavior but is self-directing in completing successive approximations toward the desired behavior until the goal is accomplished.

Modeling involves the therapist demonstrating the action to be taught to the client, either alone or simultaneously with the client through mirroring. Moore and Mathenius (1987) investigated the effects of different modeling techniques on the beat steadiness of eight adolescents with moderate mental retardation while dancing or playing a rhythm instrument. Their results indicated that, with simultaneous modeling, subjects were better able to maintain beat steadiness, though these effects were not evident in the dance condition.

Operant techniques for increasing behaviors include positive reinforcement (social approval, tangible objects, or preferred activities termed the *Premack Principle*), contracting, group contingencies, negative reinforcement, and natural reinforcement. *Positive reinforcement* is the contingent presentation of a stimulus following a response that increases the future probability of the response. Research on the contingent use of music is prevalent. In a landmark undertaking, Standley (1996) performed a meta-analysis on the effects of music as reinforcement. In all, Standley analyzed 98 studies and found highly positive results. Of the 98 studies, only 12 yielded negative effect sizes where the alternative form of reinforcement was more effective than the music. Results also indicated that music reinforcement yielded a much larger effect size than social or tangible forms of reinforcement typically used in the classroom.

The research literature reveals that contingent use of music has been used to modify behaviors ranging from improving math scores (Madsen & Forsythe, 1973; Miller, Dorow, & Greer, 1974; Yarbrough, Charboneau, & Wapnick, 1977), to developing functional speech (Talkington & Hall, 1970; Walker, 1972), and increasing attentiveness (Madsen & Alley, 1979). Researchers have also found music to be more efficacious than primary reinforcers (Saperston, Chan, Morphew, & Carsrud, 1980) and have compared differences between various levels of music reinforcement (Holloway, 1980). Other therapeutic uses of this technique include music to increase nonnutritive sucking and increase feeding rate of premature infants learning to nipple feed (Standley, 2003); music to reinforce crawling (Holliday, 1987) and head posture of children with cerebral palsy (Wolfe, 1980); music to teach acceptance of special children in an inclusive music classroom (Jellison, Brooks, & Huck, 1984); music to teach reading to Head Start children (Steele, 1971); music to reduce stereotyped behaviors (Jorgenson, 1971); music to teach auditory discrimination skills (Madsen & Geringer, 1976); music to reinforce physical therapy-directed bike pedaling for rehabilitation patients (Kendelhardt, 2003) and heel strikes of children with autism who toe walk (Roberts, 2002); music to reinforce work production in a sheltered workshop (Bellamy & Sontag, 1973; Clegg, 1982); music to reduce crying of infants with colic (Etscheidt, 1989); music to reduce EMG tension for persons with chronic headaches (Epstein, Hersen, & Hemphill, 1974); music to increase vasoconstriction of profoundly handicapped children (Falb, 1982); and music to reinforce chair sitting in order to decrease wandering of Alzheimer's patients with Sundowners syndrome (Scruggs, 1991).

Behavioral teachers and therapists provide high levels of systematic reinforcement resulting in their clients and students being more on-task in learning situations. Madsen and Alley (1979) observed 1,708 teachers and therapists and found that those who were behaviorally trained provided large, equal amounts of verbal reinforcement (83%) and achieved a correspondingly low rate of off-task behavior in their students (23% off-task for therapists and 24.8% off-task for teachers). Music and general educators who were not behaviorally trained spent far less time giving verbal reinforcement (7.6% and 7.5%, respectively), and their student off-task behavior varied concomitantly with rates of 49.3% and 56.4%, respectively.

Once established, the reinforcement is gently thinned until the newly established contingencies are no longer necessary. The effectiveness of these contingencies and efficacy of the thinning can be determined only by continued observation and recording of behavior. Johnson and Zinner (1974) demonstrated this procedure in a study to increase on-task behavior. Implementing a combination of fading and a token economy, the authors measured the responses of two young males with mental retardation. Subjects were given tokens for units of time that they were in their seat and for each unit of time that they refrained from verbalizing. These tokens could be exchanged for time listening to music or playing the piano. Gradually, the criteria for receiving tokens were increased until it was no longer possible to earn any further tokens. The authors found that the students' on-task behaviors increased when the program began, and that the level maintained even when the criteria for reward were increased and when the rewards were no longer present. As clinicians, music therapists must be concerned with generalization of the new skills and behaviors that are attained in the therapy setting and the maintenance of these behaviors outside of therapy. Johnson and Zinner illustrate the necessity of fading contrived forms of reinforcement in favor of natural reinforcement and emphasize that this is a necessary and intrinsic aspect of the therapeutic process.

Research studies often combine music and social approval to increase the probability of client success, especially if the client is severely impaired. This combination proved highly effective in Dorow's (1980) study teaching a child with mental retardation to follow directions. When compared with social approval, music is often found to be more effective. Silliman and French (1993) used contingent music versus contingent verbal approval to teach adolescents with developmental delays to kick a soccer ball. Results showed that music was more effective than either approval or music/approval combined.

The *Premack Principle* is the use of high-occurrence stimuli to reinforce low-occurrence behaviors. The elegance of this technique is that the reinforcing activity already occurs with a high frequency. Talkington and Hall (1970) applied the principle to teaching a group of 21 low-verbal individuals with mental retardation. Participants in three groups were asked to repeat words from a list of 200 items with the total number of correct repetitions tabulated. The first group was allowed to participate in 5 minutes of their most preferred musical activity if their number of correct responses was higher than in the previous session. Group two was allowed to participate in 5 minutes of their least preferred musical activity. A third group acted as a control and did not participate in music activities. The group participating in their most preferred activity had significantly more correct responses than either of the other groups. Music participation is a highly desirable and effective Premack activity. Carroccio, Lathom, and Carroccio (1976) demonstrated that contingent guitar playing aided an institutionalized mental health patient to increase periods of time without engaging in stereotypic rituals.

A *generalized conditioned reinforcer* (generalized reinforcer) is one that provides access to other types of reinforcement that can be either primary or secondary type. A clear example of this is point/token systems that, in and of themselves, possess no value but allow a person access to many other things, including activities. Dileo (1975) investigated the effects of the implementation of a token economy on the behaviors of institutionalized clients with mental retardation using musical and nonmusical rewards. Dilco also used a technique called *response cost*, wherein an undesirable behavior resulted in the removal of tokens. A chi-square analysis revealed that problem behaviors were greatly reduced as a result of the token economy and response-cost system. No data were reported regarding which of the rewards the clients selected most frequently.

Salzberg and Greenwald (1977) used a token economy without response-cost in a class of normally developing seventh-grade string students. In this study, each student was given tokens for on-task participation and punctuality to class. An invitation to a class party was the only available reward. Data showed a tremendous increase in both on-task behavior and punctuality. The authors noted that the token economy is an excellent means by which music therapists may more easily work with multiple clients of disparate functionality.

Eisenstein (1974) combined music as a contingency with a token economy system to improve the reading skills of a group of third-grade children. Each correct response when reading from flash cards or a book earned points traded for minutes of individual guitar lessons. The results indicated that those students receiving the contingency had significantly more correct reading responses.

Contracting is the placement of a contingency for reinforcement into a written document. The contract itself becomes a permanent record to which the therapist and client can refer for answering questions or avoiding uncertainties. This is particularly helpful with clients who manipulate the therapeutic situation by questioning details. Tangible, activity, and generalized reinforcers are commonly used in contracts, while social reinforcers are rarely used. If the goal is behavior management through naturally occurring reinforcement in the environment, then the therapist pairs social reinforcement with the contracted rewards. Eventually the contracted contingency, as well as the contract, becomes unnecessary.

Group contingencies can be a strong means of managing client behavior. Peer pressure plays an important role in people's lives, especially young people, so therapeutic emphasis must be placed on pressure leading toward the common good. In a classic example of this technique, Hanser (1974) successfully used group contingent music listening to reduce disruptive classroom behavior in a group of three boys with emotional disabilities. In the experiment, the boys were told that if any one person acted out, the music would stop until appropriate behavior was displayed for 15 seconds. Through several phases, inappropriate motor behaviors were decreased from 90% to 13%, while inappropriate verbal behaviors were decreased from 82% to 7%. In a similar experiment, McCarty et al. (1978) used contingent music to decrease inappropriate behavior of students with behavior disorders riding on a bus.

Negative reinforcement is the contingent removal of an aversive stimulus following a behavior that increases the future probability of the response reoccurring. An example of this might be instruction given to an adolescent with an eating disorder: "Jill, you must stay in your hospital room until you have eaten all of your food." The aversive condition (staying in the room with no stimuli for entertainment such as TV, music, books), will be removed when she has eaten the prescribed amount of food. Eating behavior is expected to increase so that she may leave the room, and it may well increase tomorrow, so that she can be with everyone else, especially if everyone is engaging in a highly preferred music activity.

Since the world often lacks consistent and contingent reinforcement schedules, it becomes important to systematically teach clients to respond to reinforcers that occur naturally as consequences of their behavior. Though one might use tokens to reward solving a problem paired with praise for a completed task, eventually the client must solve problems because it is reinforcing, or problem-solving behavior will cease at the conclusion of therapy. Reinforcers that are natural outgrowths of client behaviors are more effective than contrived reinforcers and are longer lasting.

Operant techniques for weakening behaviors include differentiated reinforcement, extinction, removal of desirable stimuli, presentation of aversive stimuli, and overcorrection. When social criteria determine that behavior is inappropriate, the classic solution to this problem is to punish. Punishment is quick and easy and works immediately. However, other more desirable techniques are available for weakening behavior. These procedures require thought and deliberation. If behaviors are to be eliminated, the desired end product that encompasses the individual behaviors of the client and the larger goal of the whole person should first be considered. If we choose a less intrusive manner to eliminate the undesirable behavior, it might take longer to extinguish, but the client might also learn appropriate behaviors for replacement. The client also maintains his or her dignity if not punished into submission.

Differentiated reinforcement is probably the least intrusive method of behavior reduction, but it works more slowly than any of the other choices. In this technique, positive reinforcement is used to increase or encourage one specified target behavior, while another targeted behavior is being reduced or eliminated. Brownell (2002) demonstrated that musically adapted social stories could provide behavioral prompts for children with autism, while simultaneously reinforcing the target behaviors of social interaction. A levels system developed by Presti (1984) systematically incorporated shaping new behaviors with differential reinforcement and consequences with the ultimate goal of generalizing new skills to the classroom and home environments.

Reinforcement of *incompatible responses* is particularly useful with clients with a large repertoire of inappropriate behaviors, often the symptom that has earned them an official diagnosis. The child with a behavior disorder may pinch, scratch, or hit other children. When reinforced to sit with his or her hands in the lap, a new behavior is taught that is incompatible with the prior problematic behavior.

Extinction is the abrupt withdrawal of positive reinforcement that is maintaining an inappropriate behavior. For example, therapists use extinction, *ignoring*, when inappropriate behavior is maintained by their attention. *Punishment* is defined as the contingent use or removal of a stimulus to decrease the occurrences of a target behavior. The term *punishment* does not occur frequently in the music therapy literature due to negative associations with the word and restrictive agency rules. Instead, operational definitions of the target behavior are stated in a positive direction to incorporate techniques for increasing, rather than decreasing behavior. Neither do music therapists typically use aversive music as a form of positive punishment, i.e., using distortion or extremely loud volume. Hanser (1987) provides an appropriate example of music as negative punishment, wherein the therapist turned off music if clients talked at an inappropriate time during a study session.

Response cost is a form of punishment in which the subject incurs a specific reduction of reinforcement (cost) for inappropriate behavior. This decreases the probability of a reoccurrence of the targeted behavior. Response cost is an attractive method of punishment for several reasons. It generally has a rapid effect on behavior, is easy to implement in a classroom setting, and can exist alongside other systems such as (and especially) a token economy. "Time out from positive reinforcement is a procedure in which access to the sources of various forms of reinforcement are removed for a particular period, contingent upon the emission of a response" (Madsen & Madsen, 1983, p. 277).

Time out is sometimes implemented by placing the misbehaving child to the side, restricting participation in the music, and prompting him or her to watch the other children for understanding of the behavior expected. This technique can also be implemented by removing the reinforcing stimuli from the client's environment. For instance, one procedure for helping adults with alcoholism who have a high attraction to spending time with their buddies in a bar is to teach the buddies to leave when their friend imbibes an alcoholic rather than a nonalcoholic beverage.

The presentation of unconditioned *aversive stimuli* that results in pain or discomfort is not recommended nor is it usually permitted within the rules of the agencies where music therapists are employed. However, conditioned (secondary) aversive stimuli merely result in social unhappiness and they are allowed.

Overcorrection involves more than one principle of behavioral change and is almost always time-consuming. The basic premise of overcorrection is that it teaches clients correct alternative behaviors in lieu of inappropriate behaviors exhibited. *Restitutional overcorrection* requires a client who has disturbed the environment by his or her misbehavior to return the setting to a state that is much improved. Juveniles who vandalize a school classroom might be required to clean all litter and graffiti and repair or replace all broken equipment. Additionally, they might be asked to paint the room, build shelves that were not previously there, and organize all equipment and materials on the new shelves.

In *positive-practice overcorrection*, the client is required to demonstrate appropriate behavior in either an exaggerated manner or overly correct practice, or for an extended period or number of times. The educative nature of positive-practice requires that the behavior assigned is the preferred alternative to the original inappropriate behavior. This technique is often used with clients in counseling to help them reduce behaviors like sarcasm (practice simple, declarative statements) or self-defeating verbalizations (practice reality-based, self-affirming verbalizations). Sometimes clients are given positive practice overcorrection assignments to complete at home between counseling visits, i.e., carrying out fixed role-playing situations such as "acting vivacious and chatty" for the individual who has difficulty meeting people. The effectiveness of this procedure demonstrates that it is easier to act one's way into a new way of thinking than to think one's way into a new way of acting (Madsen & Madsen, 1998).

Negative practice requires the client to perform the inappropriate or undesirable behavior repeatedly until satiation occurs. Fatigue causes loss of interest in continuing the inappropriate behavior. When the undesirable behavior is a response to a strong emotion, the repeated cuing of the emotion is continued until satiation occurs and the person no longer emits the response. This flooding technique is often used with persons who have grieved for very long periods of time (years) with detrimental results, such as withdrawal from family and work relationships. When the client indicates a willingness to move on with life, then the grief is cued repeatedly in one extended session through use of music that evokes memories, through use of mementos of the trauma, and through discussion of the event causing the grief. When satiation of the emotional response occurs, the person will be able to discuss the event with no withdrawal, no grief responses, and no strong emotional reaction. Flooding is widely used with crisis/rescue personnel who regularly participate in traumatic situations via an established protocol called Critical Incident Stress Treatment. It was extensively used in New York after September 11, 2001 with rescue, mortuary, and medical professionals in order to prevent the development of debilitating responses to memories of their work (Levenson & Acosta, 2001; Peterson, Nicolas, McGraw, Englert, & Blackman, 2002; Rowan, 2002).

Cognitive-Behavioral Techniques

Cognitive-behavioral techniques are used in counseling situations combining the operant procedures discussed above with techniques designed to alter cognitive perceptions essential to therapeutic success. Counseling problems are not considered pathological but rather environmental interaction problems of living. It is assumed that both prosocial and deviant behaviors are acquired and maintained in the same way and can therefore be modified similarly. In this approach, therapists assess determinants of current behavior, not its historical antecedents. Treatment plans are then individually designed based on the client's characteristics and behavior patterns, a priori analysis of the problem into its component parts (similar to task analysis), and interventions targeted at specific components. It is not necessary for clients to understand the etiology of a problem to choose other options and change their behavior. Cognitive-behavioral counseling techniques encompass the three domains of emotional distress (McGinn & Sanderson, 2001. The cognitive domain utilizes cognitive restructuring such as thought stopping or cognitive reframing, imagery, and use of evidence-based treatment manuals for consistent intervention. The behavioral domain includes exposure (flooding, desensitization), response prevention, contingency procedures such as tokens or contracts, activity scheduling, psychoeducation (problem solving, adult social skills, diagnosis/medication management issues, and assertiveness training), modeling, self-monitoring, role-playing, anger management, and behavioral activation. The physiological domain includes biofeedback and relaxation.

Cognitive-behavioral techniques are elegant therapeutic solutions, very effective in alleviating the client's distress, and therefore efficient since resolution of the problem occurs in a short period of time, which reduces therapy costs. Due to research documentation of highly successful outcomes, the cognitive-behavioral approach is the therapy of choice for anxiety disorders such as phobias and obsessive-compulsive behaviors, eating disorders, sexual disorders, and posttraumatic stress disorders (Cottraux et al., 2000; Nathan & Gorman, 2002; Turk, Fresco, & Heimberg, 1999). It is also widely used to treat depression and suicidal ideation (Hendricks, 2001). Research has shown increased benefits when music is added to progressive relaxation techniques (Scheufele, 2000) and cognitive behavior group interventions (Hendricks, 2001).

Cognitive-behavioral research literature demonstrates applications of music therapy and the above techniques. Wolfe (2000) provides a summary of cognitive-behavioral music therapy clinical treatment for short-term acute mental health settings.

A recent systematic review of psychotherapy procedures cited music therapy as an effective technique for alleviating symptoms of dementia (Livingston, Johnston, Katona, Paton, & Lyketsos, 2005). In a geriatric setting, Ashida (2000) used familiar music as a *behavior activator* to cue reminiscence in elderly persons with dementia and demonstrated reduction in depression indicators. Depression is a chronic problem for patients with dementia, though it is difficult to treat since patients cannot readily interact with the therapist. Van de Winckel, Feys, and De Weerdt (2004) used a music activity program with exercises with dementia patients and demonstrated significantly improved cognition.

Hendricks (2001) used cognitive behavioral music therapy to decrease depression symptoms in adolescents and demonstrated that music therapy in cognitive behavioral group therapy was more effective than cognitive behavioral therapy alone. He surmised that adolescents responded to the music therapy approach since music was an integral part of their life. Music therapy within group psychotherapy has also been documented as effective for adults with mental illness (de l'Etoile, 2002).

In the field of medicine, Presner et al. (2001) demonstrated that a sequenced music therapy intervention for burn patients undergoing debridement significantly reduced their perceived pain. The procedure relied upon preferred music listening followed by *progressive relaxation* then *imagery* for focus of attention away from the aversive medical procedure. Reilly (2000) used music with cataract surgery patients and demonstrated reduced blood pressure and serum cortisol levels.

Lasswell (2001) used music-assisted relaxation techniques to improve sleep quality for battered women in an abuse shelter. Sleep deprivation due to stress is a common problem that causes those in the shelter to have greater difficulty in problem solving to resolve their crisis.

Music-assisted relaxation is commonly used in medical and crisis settings to alleviate stress that complicates treatment and leads to long-term health problems. Pellitier (2004) conducted a meta-analysis that showed that both music alone and music assisted-relaxation procedures significantly decreased measures of stress. Hilliard (2001) described cognitive-behavioral procedures for counseling adolescents with eating disorders. Techniques included progressive relaxation to reduce the stress leading to the compulsion to purge, and *cognitive restructuring* to alter the cognitive distortions that caused the clients to perceive themselves as overweight. Kerr, Walsh, and Marshall (2001) combined music with *cognitive-reframing* interventions and demonstrated this treatment was more effective than cognitive-reframing alone. Subjects were anxious adults who demonstrated significant reductions in anxiety measures, increased modification in affect, and increased vividness of imagery. Sundar (2006) reported using psychoeducation and music therapy to assist a cancer patient in managing distress and situational anxiety related to treatment. Following a review of the empirical data in hospice research and music therapy, Hilliard (2005) concluded that music therapy alleviated anxiety and positively affected pain, physical comfort, duration of treatment, and quality of life for those with terminal illnesses.

In 2002, Gallagher and Steele described a comprehensive cognitive-behavioral music therapy clinical model for treatment of those with substance abuse problems and reported effective results. Jones (2005) demonstrated that music therapy interventions utilizing song writing and lyric analysis evoked significant emotional changes in chemically dependent clients. On their discharge questionnaires, the clients also strongly indicated that music therapy was perceived as an important part of their treatment process. Dingle, Gleadhill, and Baker (2008) combined music therapy with a 7-week cognitive behavioral treatment for substance abuse. They found that attendance to sessions was high and that patients reported high levels of engagement and enjoyment. Music therapy for emotion exploration has also been proven an effective cognitive-behavioral methodology for those with substance abuse problems (Baker, Gleadhill, & Dingle, 2007), as has activity-based behavioral activation music therapy (Cevasco, Kennedy, & Generally, 2005).

DeBedout (1994) showed that music activities and focused discussion assisted juveniles in court-mandated detention with values clarification issues. The music activities significantly improved positive value statements. James (1988) demonstrated that song lyric analysis contributed to values clarification and increased the perceived locus of control of adolescents in rehabilitation for chemical dependency.

Clinical programs in cognitive behavioral music therapy have been used to reduce burnout symptoms in teachers (Cheek, Bradley, Parr, & Lan, 2003) and nurses (Watanabe, 2001) and to assist trauma survivors. Slatoroff (1994) reported on use of improvisational drumming techniques for teaching *assertiveness and anger management*. This cognitive behavioral approach was designed to offset trauma for adults and adolescents who were victims of rape, natural disasters, violent crime, childhood abuse, and domestic violence.

Cassity's (2006) Delphi poll revealed the prediction that psychoeducation was becoming a more important aspect of psychiatric music therapy for the future. Psychiatric patients perceive music therapy for psychoeducation to be an important to their treatment (Silverman, 2006). In 2007, Silverman (2007a) demonstrated the benefits of a single cognitive-behavioral music therapy session utilizing a psychoeducational treatment manual for psychiatric patients. His dependent measures were varied across quality of life, knowledge of illness, and treatment perceptions. Perhaps most importantly, he developed an innovative method for observing group therapy verbalizations and assessing degree of insight in the group discussion content.

Status of Behavioral Research in Music Therapy

The techniques discussed above and research nested within each section, along with the extensive body of research available to music therapists, provide a strong foundation of efficacy of the behavioral approach. As the clinical use of the behavioral model continues to stimulate applied research, music therapists will build resources to demonstrate the viability not only of this particular methodology, but music therapy in general. Cognitive-behavioral music therapy is an evidence-based approach that meets the highest standards of professional practice in psychotherapy.

Conclusion

Behaviorism is a field of psychology that has had a widely accepted presence throughout our culture. The advent of behavioral practices had a notable impact on educational and health systems at every level. Scientifically, applied behavior analysis stimulated a dramatic increase in quantity and quality of treatment research. As a result of this burgeoning research, clinical practitioners have been presented with clearly delineated and replicable methodologies for the treatment of real patients (Wilson, 2000).

Music therapy was not involved in the initial manifestations of behaviorism; however, the profession did adopt behavioral techniques early on. One principal reason was how easily and effectively the techniques fit into a music therapy paradigm. The techniques discussed in this chapter can greatly enhance music therapy interventions when used appropriately. Client behavior at all age levels can be targeted, observed, and moved in a positive direction in psychotherapy for all types of problems. Also integral to many music therapy settings, behaviorism allows both cognitive and affective domains to be therapeutically treated.

As the demand for accountability and therapeutic impact continues to increase from third-party payers as well as consumers, the objective evidence of treatment effectiveness becomes even more consequential. Many predict that due to increasing health costs, psychotherapies will be subjected to increased scrutiny by third-party payers and perhaps face a critical period of denial for reimbursement. It is also predicted that therapists using accountability methods with proven, empirically documented outcomes of client improvement will flourish.

References

Alberto, P. A., & Troutman, A. C. (1995). *Applied behavior analysis for teachers* (4th ed.). Englewood Cliffs, NJ: Merrill.

Ashida, S. (2000). The effect of reminiscence music therapy sessions on changes in depressive symptoms in elderly persons with dementia. *Journal of Music Therapy, 37*, 170–195.

Ayllon, T., & Michael, J. (1959). The psychiatric nurse as a behavioral engineer. *Journal of the Experimental Analysis of Behavior, 2*, 323–334.

Baars, B. J. (1986). *The cognitive revolution in psychology*. New York: Guilford Press.

Baker, F., Gleadhill, L., & Dingle, G. (2007). Music therapy and emotional exploration: Exposing substance abuse clients to the experiences of non-drug-induced emotions. *The Arts in Psychotherapy, 34, 321–330.*

Bandura, A. (1969). *Principles of behavior modification*. San Francisco: Holt, Rinehart, and Winston.

Bellamy, T., & Sontag, E. (1973). Use of group contingent music to increase assembly line production rates of retarded students in a simulated sheltered workshop. *Journal of Music Therapy, 10*, 125–136.

Bergin, A. E., & Garfield, S. L. (1994). *Handbook of psychotherapy and behavior change*. New York: J. Wiley.

Brownell, M. D. (2002). Musically adapted social stories to modify behaviors in students with autism: Four case studies. *Journal of Music Therapy, 39,* 117–144.

Bryant, D. R. (1987). A cognitive approach to therapy through music. *Journal of Music Therapy, 24,* 27–34.

Carroccio, D. F., Latham, S., & Carroccio, B. B. (1976). Rate-contingent guitar rental to decelerate stereotyped head/face-touching of an adult male psychiatric patient. *Behavior Therapy, 7*, 104–109.

Cassity, M. (2006). *Psychiatric music therapy in 2016: A Delphi poll of the future.* Paper presented at the annual conference of the American Music Therapy Association, Kansas City, MO.

Cevasco, A., Kennedy, R., & Generally, N. (2005). Comparison of movement-to-music, rhythm activities, and competitive games on depression, stress, anxiety, and anger of females in substance abuse rehabilitation. *Journal of Music Therapy, 42,* 64–80.

Cheek, J. R., Bradley, L. J., Parr, G., & Lan, W. (2003). Using music therapy techniques to treat teacher burnout. *Journal of Mental Health Counseling, 25,* 204–217.

Clair, A. A. (1996). *Therapeutic uses of music with older adults.* Baltimore: Health Professions Press.

Clegg, J. C. (1982). *The effect of non-contingent and contingent music on work production rate of mentally retarded adults in a work activity center.* Unpublished master's thesis, Florida State University, Tallahassee.

Cooper, J. O., Heron, T. E., & Heward, W. L. (1987). *Applied behavior analysis.* New York: Macmillan.

Cottraux, J., Note, I., Albuisson, E., Yao, S. N., Note, B., Mollard, E., Bonasse, F., Jalenques, I., Guerin, J., & Coudert, A. J. (2000). Cognitive behavior therapy versus supportive therapy in social phobia: A randomized controlled trial. *Psychotherapy & Psychosomatics, 69,* 137–146.

Darrow, A., Gfeller, K., Gorsuch, A., Thomas, K. (2000). Music therapy with children who are deaf and hard of hearing. In American Music Therapy Association (Ed.), *Effectiveness of music therapy procedures: Documentation of research and clinical practice.* Silver Spring, MD: American Music Therapy Association.

Davis, C. A. (1992). The effects of music and basic relaxation instruction on pain and anxiety in women undergoing in-office gynecological procedures. *Journal of Music Therapy, 29,* 202–216.

Davis, W. B., Gfeller, K. E., & Thaut, M. H. (2008). *An introduction to music therapy: Theory and practice* (3rd ed.). Dubuque, IA: McGraw Hill.

DeBedout, J. K. (1994). *The effect of music activity versus a non-music activity on verbalization and values clarification during group counseling with juvenile offenders.* Unpublished master's thesis, Florida State University, Tallahassee.

de l'Etoile, S. (2002). The effectiveness of music therapy in group psychotherapy for adults with mental illness. *The Arts in Psychotherapy, 29,* 69–78.

Dileo, C. L. (1975). The use of a token economy program with mentally retarded persons in a music therapy setting. *Journal of Music Therapy, 12,* 155–160.

Dingle, G. A., Gleadhill, L. & Baker, F. A. (2008). Can music therapy engage patients in group cognitive behaviour therapy for substance abuse treatment? *Drug and Alcohol Review, 27*(2), 190–196.

Dorow, L. G. (1975). Conditioning music and approval as new reinforcers for imitative behavior with the severely retarded. *Journal of Music Therapy, 12,* 30–39.

Dorow, L. G. (1980). Generalization effects of newly conditioned reinforcers. *Journal of Music Therapy, 15,* 8–14.

Eifert, G. H., & Plaud, J. J. (1998). From behavior theory to behavior therapy: An overview. In J. J. Plaud & G. H. Eifert (Eds.), *From behavior theory to behavior therapy* (pp. 1–14). Boston: Allyn and Bacon.

Eisenstein, S. R. (1974). Effect of contingent guitar lessons on reading behavior. *Journal of Music Therapy, 11,* 138–146.

Eisenstein, S. R. (1976). A successive approximation procedure for learning music symbol names. *Journal of Music Therapy, 13,* 173–179.

Ellis, A. (1987). The use of rational humorous songs in psychotherapy. In W. F. Fry, Jr., & W. A. Salameh (Eds.), *Handbook of humor and psychotherapy* (pp. 265–285). Sarasota, FL: Professional Resource Exchange.

Ellis, A. (2003). *A garland of rational songs.* Audiotape distributed by Albert Ellis Institute. www.rebt.org

Epstein, L., Hersen, M., & Hemphill, D. (1974). Music feedback in the treatment of tension headache: An experimental case study. *Journal of Behavioral Therapy and Experimental Psychiatry, 5,* 59–63.

Etscheidt, M. A. (1989). *Parent training to reduce excessive crying associated with infant colic.* Unpublished doctoral dissertation, Georgia State University, Atlanta.

Falb, M. E. (1982). *The use of operant procedures to condition vasoconstriction in profoundly mentally retarded (PMR) infants.* Unpublished master's thesis, Florida State University, Tallahassee.

Fuller, P. R. (1949). Operant conditioning of a vegetative organism. *American Journal of Psychology, 62,* 587–590.

Gallagher, L. M., & Steele, A. L. (2002). Music therapy with offenders in a substance abuse/mental illness treatment program. *Music Therapy Perspectives, 20*(2), 117–122.

Gaston, E. T. (1968). *Music in therapy.* New York: Macmillan.

Gfeller, K. E. (1987). Music therapy theory and practice as reflected in research literature. *Journal of Music Therapy, 24,* 178–194.

Ghetti, C. M. (2002). Comparison of the effectiveness of three music therapy conditions to modulate behavior states in students with profound disabilities: A pilot study. *Music Therapy Perspectives, 20,* 20–30.

Gilliland, E. G. (1962). Progress in music therapy. *Rehabilitation Literature, 23,* 298–306.

Gregory, D. (2002). Four decades of music therapy behavioral research designs: A content analysis of *Journal of Music Therapy* articles. *Journal of Music Therapy, 39,* 56–71.

Hanser, S. B. (1974). Group-contingent music listening with emotionally disturbed boys. *Journal of Music Therapy, 11,* 220–225.

Hanser, S. B. (1983). Music therapy: A behavioral perspective. *The Behavior Therapist, 6,* 5–8.

Hanser, S. B. (1987). Stage 5: Determining music therapy strategies. In *Music therapist's handbook* (pp. 103–125). St. Louis, MO: Warren H. Green.

Hanser, S. B. (1990). A music therapy strategy for depressed older adults in the community. *Journal of Applied Gerontology, 9,* 283–298.

Hanser, S. B. (1995). Applied behavior analysis. In B. L. Wheeler (Ed.), *Music therapy research: Quantitative and qualitative perspectives* (pp. 149–164). Phoenixville, PA: Barcelona.

Hendricks, C. B. (2001). A study of the use of music therapy techniques in a group for the treatment of adolescent depression. *Dissertation Abstracts International, 62*(2-A), 472.

Hilliard, R. E. (2001). The use of cognitive-behavioral music therapy in the treatment of women with eating disorders. *Music Therapy Perspectives, 19,* 109–113.

Hilliard, R. E. (2005). Music therapy in Hospice and palliative care: A review of the empirical data. *Evidence-based Complementary and Alternative Medicine, 2*(2), 173–178. Retrieved April 29, 2008, from http://ecam.oxfordjournals.org/cgi/content/full/2/2/173

Holliday, A. M. (1987). *Music therapy and physical therapy to habilitate physical disabilities of young children*. Unpublished master's thesis, Florida State University, Tallahassee.

Holloway, M. S. (1980). A comparison of passive and active music reinforcement to increase preacademic and motor skills in severely retarded children and adolescents. *Journal of Music Therapy, 17,* 58–69.

James, M. (1988). Music therapy values clarification: A positive influence on perceived locus of control. *Journal of Music Therapy, 25*(4), 206–215.

Jellison, J. A., Brooks, B., & Huck, A. (1984). Structuring small groups and music reinforcement to facilitate positive interactions and acceptance of severely handicapped students in the regular music classroom. *Journal of Research in Music Education, 32,* 243–264.

Johnson, J. M., & Zinner, C. C. (1974). Stimulus fading and schedule learning in generalizing and maintaining behaviors. *Journal of Music Therapy, 11,* 84–86.

Jones, J. D. (2005). A comparison of songwriting and lyric analysis techniques to evoke emotional change in a single session with people who are chemically dependent. *Journal of Music Therapy, 42,* 94–110.

Jorgenson, H. (1971). Effects of contingent preferred music in reducing two stereotyped behaviors of a profoundly retarded child. *Journal of Music Therapy, 8,* 139–145.

Kendelhardt, A. R. (2003). *The effect of live music on exercise duration, negative verbalizations, and self-perception of pain, anxiety, and rehabilitation levels of physical therapy patients*. Unpublished master's thesis, Florida State University, Tallahassee.

Kerr, T., Walsh, J., & Marshall, A. (2001). Emotional change processes in music-assisted reframing. *Journal of Music Therapy, 38,* 193–211.

Krasner, L., & Ullman, L. P. (1965). *Research in behavior modification: New developments and implications*. New York: Holt, Rinehart, and Winston.

Lasswell, A. R. (2001). *The effects of music assisted relaxation on the relaxation, sleep quality, and daytime sleepiness of sheltered, abused women*. Unpublished master's thesis, Florida State University, Tallahassee.

Levenson, R. L., Jr., & Acosta, J. K. (2001). Observations from Ground Zero at the World Trade Center in New York City, Part I. *International Journal of Emergency Mental Health, 3,* 241–244.

Livingston, G., Johnston, K., Katona, C., Paton, J., & Lyketsos, C. (2005). Systematic review of psychological approaches to the management of neuropsychiatric symptoms of dementia. *American Journal of Psychiatry, 162,* 1996–2021.

Madsen, C. H., & Madsen, C. K. (1983). *Teaching/Discipline: A positive approach for educational development* (3rd ed.). Raleigh, NC: Contemporary.

Madsen, C. K. (1999, November). *A behavioral approach to music therapy*. Founding Model Address to the General Assembly, 9th World Congress of Music Therapy, Washington, DC.

Madsen, C. K., & Alley, J. M. (1979). The effect of reinforcement on attentiveness: A comparison of behaviorally trained music therapists and other professionals with implications for competency-based academic preparation. *Journal of Music Therapy, 16,* 70–82.

Madsen, C. K., & Forsythe, J. L. (1973). Effect of contingent music listening on increases in mathematical response. *Journal of Research in Music Education, 21,* 176–181.

Madsen, C. K., & Geringer, J. (1976). Choice of televised music lessons versus free play in relationship to academic improvement. *Journal of Music Therapy, 13,* 154–162.

Madsen, C. K., & Madsen, C. H. (1968). Music as a behavior modification technique with a juvenile delinquent. *Journal of Music Therapy, 3,* 72–76.

Madsen, C. K., & Madsen, C. H. (1998). *Teaching/Discipline: A positive approach for educational development* (4th ed.). Raleigh, NC: Contemporary.

Mandel, S. E. (1996). Music for wellness: Music therapy for stress management in a rehabilitation program. *Music Therapy Perspectives, 14,* 38–43.

Masters, J. C., Burish, T. G., Hollon, S. D., & Rimm, D. C. (1987). *Behavior therapy: Techniques and empirical findings* (3rd ed.). San Diego, CA: Harcourt Brace Jovanovich.

Maultsby, M. C. (1977). Combining music therapy and rational behavior therapy. *Journal of Music Therapy, 14,* 89–97.

McCarthy, K. M. (1992). Stress management in the health care field: A pilot program for staff in a nursing home unit for patients with Alzheimer's disease. *Music Therapy Perspectives, 10,* 110–113.

McCarty, B. C., McElfresh, C. T., Rice, S. V., & Wilson, S. J. (1978). The effect of contingent background music on inappropriate bus behavior. *Journal of Music Therapy, 15,* 150–156.

McGinn, L. K., & Sanderson, W.C. (2001). What allows cognitive behavioral therapy to be brief: Overview, efficacy, and crucial factors facilitating brief treatment. *Clinical Psychology: Science and Practice, 8*(1), 23–37.

Miller, D. M., Dorow, L., & Greer, R. D. (1974). The contingent use of music and art for improving arithmetic scores. *Journal of Music Therapy, 11,* 57–64.

Moore, R., & Mathenius, L. (1987). The effects of modeling, reinforcement, and tempo on imitative rhythmic response of moderately retarded adolescents. *Journal of Music Therapy, 24,* 160–169.

Nathan, P. E. (Ed.), & Gorman, J. M. (2002). *A guide to treatments that work* (2nd ed.). New York: Oxford University Press.

Pelletier, C. L. (2004). The effect of music on decreasing arousal due to stress: A meta-analysis. *Journal of Music Therapy, 41*(3), 192–214.

Peterson, A. L., Nicolas, M. G., McGraw, K., Englert, D., & Blackman, L. R. (2002). Psychological intervention with mortuary workers after the September 11 attack: The Dover Behavioral Health Consultant Model. *Military Medicine, 167,* 83–86.

Presner, J., Fratianne, R., Yowler, C., Standley, J., Steele, L., & Smith, L. (2001). The effect of music based imagery and musical alternate engagement on the burn debridement process. *Journal of Burn Care and Rehabilitation, 22,* 47–53.

Presti, G. M. (1984). A levels system approach to music therapy with severely behaviorally handicapped children in the public school system. *Journal of Music Therapy, 21,* 117–125.

Reilly, M. P. (2000). Music, a cognitive behavioral intervention for anxiety and acute pain control in the elderly cataract patient. *Dissertation Abstracts International, 60*(7-B), 3195.

Rider, M. S., Floyd, J. W., & Kirkpatrick, J. (1985). The effect of music, imagery, and relaxation on adrenal corticosteroids and the re-entrainment of circadian rhythms. *Journal of Music Therapy, 22,* 46–58.

Robb, S. L. (2000). The effect of therapeutic music interventions on the behavior of hospitalized children in isolation: Developing a contextual support model of music therapy. *Journal of Music Therapy, 37,* 118–146.

Robb, S. L., Nichols, R. J., Rutan, R. L., Bishop, B. L., & Parker, J. C. (1995). The effects of music assisted relaxation on preoperative anxiety. *Journal of Music Therapy, 17*, 2–15.

Roberts, P. (2002). *The effect of contingent music with physical therapy in children who toe-walk.* Unpublished master's thesis, Florida State University, Tallahassee.

Rowan, A. B. (2002). Air Force Critical Incident Stress Management Outreach with Pentagon staff after the terrorist attack. *Military Medicine, 197*, 33–35.

Salzberg, R. S., & Greenwald, M. A. (1977). Effects of a token system of attentiveness and punctuality in two string instrument classes. *Journal of Music Therapy, 14*, 27–38.

Saperston, B. M., Chan, R., Morphew, C., & Carsrud, K. B. (1980). Music listening versus juice as a reinforcement for learning in profoundly mentally retarded individuals. *Journal of Music Therapy, 17*, 174–183.

Scartelli, J. P. (1984). The effect of EMG biofeedback and sedative music, EMG biofeedback only, and sedative music only on frontalis muscle relaxation ability. *Journal of Music Therapy, 21*, 67–78.

Scheufele, P. M. (2000). Effects of progressive relaxation and classical music on measurements of attention, relaxation, and stress responses. *Journal of Behavioral Medicine, 23*, 207–228.

Scovel, M. A. (1990). Music therapy within the context of psychotherapeutic models. In R. F. Unkefer (Ed.), *Music therapy in the treatment of adults with mental disorders* (pp. 96–108). New York: Schirmer Books.

Scruggs, S. D. (1991). *The effects of structured music activities versus contingent music listening with verbal prompt on wandering behavior and cognition in geriatric patients with Alzheimer's disease.* Unpublished master's thesis, Florida State University, Tallahassee.

Sears, W. W. (1968). Processes in music therapy. In E. T. Gaston (Ed.), *Music in therapy* (pp. 30–44). New York: Macmillan.

Selm, M. E. (1991). Chronic pain: Three issues in treatment and implications for music therapy. *Music Therapy Perspectives, 9*, 91–97.

Silliman, L. M., & French, R. (1993). Use of selected reinforcers to improve the ball kicking of youths with profound mental retardation. *Adapted Physical Activity Quarterly, 10*, 52–69.

Silverman, M. J. (2006). Psychiatric patients' perception of music therapy and other psychoeducational programming. *Journal of Music Therapy, 43*, 111–122.

Silverman, M. J. (2007a). *The effect of single-session psychoeducational music therapy on response frequency and type, satisfaction with life, knowledge of illness, and treatment perceptions in psychiatric patients.* Unpublished doctoral dissertation, Florida State University, Tallahassee.

Silverman, M. J. (2007b). Evaluating current trends in psychiatric music therapy: A descriptive analysis. *Journal of Music Therapy, 44*(4), 388–414.

Skinner, B. F. (1948). *Walden two.* London: Macmillan.

Skinner, B. F. (1953). *Science and human behavior.* New York: Macmillan.

Slateroff, C. (1994). Drumming technique for assertiveness and anger management in the short-term psychiatric setting for adult and adolescent survivors of trauma. *Music Therapy Perspectives, 12*(1), 111–116.

Standley, J. M. (1996). A meta-analysis on the effects of music as reinforcement for education/therapy objectives. *Journal of Research in Music Education, 44*, 105–133.

Standley, J. M. (1998). The effect of music and multimodal stimulation on physiologic and developmental responses of premature infants in neonatal intensive care. *Pediatric Nursing, 21*, 532–539.

Standley, J. M. (2003). The effect of music-reinforced non-nutritive sucking on feeding rate of premature infants. *Journal of Pediatric Nursing, 18,* 169–173.

Steele, A. L. (1971). Contingent socio-music listening periods in a preschool setting. *Journal of Music Therapy, 8,* 131–139.

Steele, A. L. (1977). The application of behavioral research techniques to community music therapy. *Journal of Music Therapy, 14,* 102–115.

Sundar, S. (2006). Effects of music therapy and counseling: A case of state anxiety of a ca-hypo pharynx patient [Electronic version]. *Music Therapy Today, 7*(1), 8–29.

Talkington, L. W., & Hall, S. M. (1970). A musical application of Premack's hypothesis to low verbal retardates. *Journal of Music Therapy, 7*, 95–99.

Thaut, M. H. (1989). Music therapy, affect modification, and therapeutic change: Towards an integrative model. *Music Therapy Perspectives, 7,* 55–62.

Turk, C. L., Fresco, D. M., & Heimberg, R. G. (1999). Cognitive behavior therapy. In M. Hersen & A. S. Bellack (Eds.), *Handbook of comparative interventions for adult disorders* (2nd ed., pp. 287–316). New York: John Wiley & Sons.

Ullman, L. P., & Krasner, L. (1965). *Case studies in behavior modification.* New York: Holt, Rinehart, and Winston.

Van de Winckel, A., Feys, H. & De Weerdt, W. (2004). Cognitive and behavioural effects of music-based exercises in patients with dementia. *Clinical Rehabilitation, 18*(3), 253–260.

Walker, J. B. (1972). The use of music as an aid in developing functional speech in the institutionalized mentally retarded. *Journal of Music Therapy, 9,* 1–12.

Watanabe, K. (2001). *The effects of music with abbreviated progressive relaxation techniques on occupational stress in female nurses in a hospital.* Unpublished master's thesis, Florida State University, Tallahassee.

Wheeler, B. (1981). The relationship between music therapy and theories of psychotherapy. *Music Therapy, 1,* 9–16.

Wilson, G. T. (2000). Behavior therapy. In R. J. Corsini & D. Wedding (Eds.), *Current psychotherapies* (6th ed., pp. 205–240). Itasca, IL: F. E. Peacock.

Wolfe, D. E. (1980). The effect of automated interrupted music on head posturing of cerebral palsied individuals. *Journal of Music Therapy, 17*, 184–206.

Wolfe, D. E. (2000). Group music therapy in acute mental health care: Meeting the demands of effectiveness and efficiency. In American Music Therapy Association (Ed.), *Effectiveness of music therapy procedures: Documentation of research and clinical practice* (pp. 265–296). Silver Spring, MD: American Music Therapy Association.

Wolfe, D. E., & Horn, C. (1993). Use of melodies as structural prompts for learning and retention of sequential verbal information by preschool clients. *Journal of Music Therapy, 30,* 100–118.

Yarbrough, C., Charboneau, M., & Wapnick, J. (1977). Music as reinforcement for correct math and attending in ability assigned math classes. *Journal of Music Therapy, 14,* 77–88.

Recommended Additional Readings

Ayllon, T., & Azrin, N. H. (1968). *The token economy: A motivational system for therapy and rehabilitation.* New York: Appleton.

Eidson, C. E. (1989). The effect of behavioral music therapy on the generalization of interpersonal skills from sessions to the classroom by emotionally handicapped middle school clients. *Journal of Music Therapy, 26,* 206–221.

Harding, C., & Ballard, K. D. (1982). The effectiveness of music as a stimulus and as a contingent reward in promoting the spontaneous speech of three physically handicapped preschoolers. *Journal of Music Therapy, 19,* 86–101.

Hauck, L. P., & Martin, P. L. (1970). Music as a reinforcer in patient-controlled duration of time-out. *Journal of Music Therapy, 7,* 43–53.

James, M. R. (1986). Verbal reinforcement and self-monitoring inclinations. *Journal of Music Therapy, 23,* 182–193.

Jorgenson, H. (1974). The use of a contingent music activity to modify behaviors, which interfere with learning. *Journal of Music Therapy, 11,* 41–46.

Madsen, C. K. (2003). *A behavioral approach to music therapy.* Retrieved September 16, 2003, from http://www.ejournal.unam.ms/clinvedmus/vol01-02/CEM02102.pdf

Madsen, C. K., Cotter, V., & Madsen, C. H., Jr. (1968). A behavioral approach to music therapy. *Journal of Music Therapy, 5,* 70–75.

McClure, J. T. (1986). Reduction of hand mouthing by a boy with profound mental retardation. *Mental Retardation, 24,* 219–222.

Reid, D. H., Hill, B. K., Rawers, R. J., & Montegar, C. A. (1975). The use of contingent music in teaching social skills to a nonverbal, hyperactive boy. *Journal of Music Therapy, 12,* 2–18.

Silverman, S. H., & Miller, F. D. (1971). The use of the Premack Principle and a buddy system in a normal eighth grade class. *SALT, 4,* 14–19.

Wilson, C. V. (1976). The use of rock music as a reward in behavior therapy with children. *Journal of Music Therapy, 13,* 39–48.

Section Three

Medical Approaches to
Music Therapy

Chapter 9

Music Therapy in Wellness

Claire Mathern Ghetti
Mika Hama
Jennifer Woolrich

Introduction

Wellness care focuses on achieving and maintaining a state of personal health by optimizing as many aspects of an individual's lifestyle and well-being as possible. Several definitions can clarify the comprehensiveness of the wellness model. Ebersole and Hess (1981) defined wellness as the creation of a homeostasis by finding an internal and external balance between emotional, social, cultural, physical, and environmental stimuli. This holistic balance is formed by the interplay of the following domains of wellness: (a) self-responsibility, (b) nutritional awareness, (c) physical fitness, (d) stress management, and (e) environmental sensitivity (Travis, 1977). These dimensions of wellness have formed the backbone of many wellness programs. Dunn (1959), one of the first wellness pioneers to emphasize the importance of the health of mind, body, and spirit, described wellness as a methodological approach that aims to maximize an individual's potential within the environment where he or she is functioning. Thus, a wellness paradigm integrates physical, mental, and spiritual aspects of being to result in a state of holistic health (Lipe, 2002).

In addition to defining wellness as a state of holistic balance, it also refers to efforts toward prevention of disease and achievement of well-being, despite the presence of illness. With the latter definition, an individual with a chronic illness may achieve a sense of wellness by managing symptoms of the illness. Experiencing high quality of life while living with illness may be achieved through modulating perceptions, illness experience, and functional status in a desired direction (Watt, Verma, & Flynn, 1998). A positive sense of well-being and improved quality of life may, in turn, enhance one's physical health. Thus, wellness behaviors and attitudes influence an individual's continuing quest for health and can positively influence illness (Benson & McDevitt, 1989).

Wellness is formally recognized as an area of music therapy practice, with the American Music Therapy Association (AMTA) defining corresponding standards of clinical practice. AMTA defines the use of music therapy in wellness as "the specialized use of music to enhance quality of life, maximize well-being and potential, and increase self-awareness in individuals seeking music therapy services" (AMTA, 2005). Thus, wellness music therapy may enhance holistic well-being and prevent illness for healthy individuals, or help promote balance and quality of life for those with chronic illnesses.

The past decade has evidenced a significant increase in research evaluating the effectiveness of music to promote wellness, as well as rapid growth of clinical applications of wellness music therapy. A significant portion of this research evaluates the effects of music therapy on neurophysiological functioning, healthy behavior patterns, and psychological health to promote immune system functioning, healthy stress management, adherence to healthy lifestyle changes, and improved mood states. Clinical techniques of wellness music therapy are diverse and include therapeutic drumming, active music making, music listening, music-based wellness exercises, movement and music programs, guided imagery and music, singing, and lyric analysis.

The wellness model has important implications for all age groups. Focusing on holistic health of older adults can increase quality of life, alleviate depression, prevent or lessen the impact of chronic stress-related diseases, and reduce the chances of hospitalized treatments that often include invasive medical procedures. Changing a high-stress lifestyle into a wellness-based lifestyle for middle-aged adults likewise helps prevent or postpone stress-related or stress-agitated conditions. Understandably, the earlier one starts a healthy lifestyle, the more benefits one will reap. Teaching children about nutrition, exercise, relaxation, and stress management may prevent health problems, improve emotional health, and even boost academic achievement (Murray, Low, Hollis, Cross, & Davis, 2007). The wellness model consists of several lifestyle components that together result in holistic health. Music therapy is one efficacious and motivating approach used to promote holistic health in a variety of population groups.

The purpose of this chapter is to explore the history and present state of wellness in various sectors of society, survey the research related to music therapy and wellness, and present a review of clinical applications of music therapy in wellness.

History of Wellness Programs

Prior to the 1970s, the role of Western allopathic medicine was limited to finding treatment and cures for diseases. Health was measured in terms of lack of disease, with physical status being the primary focus. If a person did not have a physical ailment, then he or she was considered to be well. Health was simply the absence of illness. Prior to the wellness movement, individuals did not consider that they could be responsible for their own health. Patients were content to hand all responsibility for restoring health to their physicians and were willing to follow their physicians' orders without question. Health was seen as something that was accessible only via knowledgeable physicians, and therefore it was something to be bought from the medical world (Edlin & Golanty, 1992).

Attitudes shifted in the late 1970s when people began to apprehend the importance of preventive efforts as a means to avoid or alleviate illness. As a result of a policy statement issued by the American Hospital Association in 1979, hospitals began developing wellness programs. Given the opportunity to participate in wellness programs, people gradually realized that implementing lifestyle changes could prevent many illnesses (Gutt, 1996).

Gutt (1996) identified several factors that contributed to the rapid growth of the wellness movement. As technology advanced, the cost of health care increased, which caused many people, including employers, to seek less expensive ways of maintaining health in order to avoid the high cost of illness. Physical fitness became a popular leisure activity, leading many people to reevaluate their lifestyles. Ecologists also began to raise concerns over environmental effects on people's health and saw a need for change. As these developments took place, medical research broadened its focus to encompass the study of the impact of wellness and lifestyle changes on health.

Although the conceptualization of health as the absence of physical illness continues to dominate, since the 1980s there has been a shift toward a holistic view that considers physical, mental, social, and spiritual aspects of health. This holistic view assumes that all the various components of health are intertwined and affect a person's well-being. As this view of holistic health gained popularity, the term *wellness* emerged to describe the comprehensive soundness of body-mind-spirit of an individual that emanates from all aspects of a person's lifestyle. Health is no longer defined by physical well-being alone.

History of Wellness Programs for Older Adults

Like other areas of medical care, health care of the older adult population in the United States has traditionally emphasized illness care. Past research investigated the effects of the disease process on aging and generally avoided examining the health of older adults. Older adults were not viewed as appropriate targets of health promotion efforts (Walker, 1991), yet illness-based care alone did not significantly increase life expectancy or improve life quality for the majority of older individuals. Beginning in the 1980s, attention began to shift among health care professionals, and interest regarding health care approaches for prevention of illness and promotion of health increased (Walker, 1991). In 1988, the U.S. Surgeon General convened the Workshop of Health Promotion and Aging to assess current knowledge on health promotion among older adults and to make recommendations for policy, service, education, and research in these areas (Walker, 1991). Such initiatives played an important role in developing the structures and support systems of a comprehensive wellness program for older adults. Wellness and prevention programs for older adults have also proven economically sound, as they are more cost-effective than illness-based care (Benson & McDevitt, 1989).

It is also important to acknowledge the efforts of holistic nursing for promoting wellness among older persons. It may be postulated that wellness programs for older adults originated in part from holistic nursing practices. Nurses who emphasize self-care and self-responsibility and provide education and opportunities in the various dimensions of wellness have helped spread the wellness lifestyle to older individuals (Wilson, Patterson, & Alford, 1989). Holistic nursing encompasses illness care in addition to wellness care; consequently, it can be viewed as a comprehensive health model. As more research is published in health care journals regarding the effects of exercise, nutrition, socialization, and other wellness dimensions on the life quality and health of older individuals, a different style of aging is emerging (Bruhn & Clair, 1999; Miller, 1991).

History of Wellness Programs in Corporations

Since the late 1970s, American businesses have faced dramatically increasing health care costs for their employees. Employee health insurance costs, medical claims, loss of productivity, and absenteeism have become serious financial burdens to employers (Jacobson et al., 1996). In 1970, health care costs were 7.5% of the gross national product (GNP); by 1990, they had risen to 12% (Anspaugh, Hunter, & Mosley, 1995; Chenoweth, 1991). Since many corporations were losing profits as a result of the increase in health care costs for their employees, businesses began to seek out cost-cutting alternatives, including health promotion or wellness programs. Many of these programs showed promise for reducing the cost of health care to both large and small companies (Anspaugh et al., 1995; Glasgow & Terborg, 1988; Goldsmith, 1986; Stokols, Pelletier, & Fielding, 1996). Because wellness programs decreased the likelihood or impact of diseases, disabilities, or both, implementing such programs for all workers decreased the cost of covering medical care expenses for employees.

In the 1980s, the number of health promotion programs in the workplace started to increase (Bulaclac, 1996; Glasgow & Terborg, 1988). Coors, the well-known beer manufacturer, opened wellness centers to provide health promotion and disease prevention programs to employees in 1981. These programs saved the company at least $1.9 million annually due to lower medical cost increases, reduced sick leave, and increased productivity (Chenoweth, 1991). J. P. Morgan Co., Inc., AT&T, and General Motors followed suit by designing comprehensive health promotion programs that successfully decreased health care costs, mortality, morbidity, number of workdays missed, on-the-job accidents, and overall lost time (Anspaugh et al., 1995). The initial reason for implementing health promotion or wellness programs in corporate settings was the desire to decrease health care costs. Although these programs were originally used as a means of combating the high costs of covering employee medical care, they turned out to have many hidden advantages for the companies that used them. Among the unexpected benefits resulting from the implementation of wellness programs were increases in employee stamina and productivity; boosting of employee morale; increased creativity in employees' work tasks; decreases in absenteeism and sick leave; increases in job satisfaction; improvement in time management, concentration, and decision-making ability; and decreased turnover rate.

It is now estimated that 90% of companies offer at least one component of a wellness program to their employees (Aldana, Merrill, Price, Hardy, & Hager, 2005). As health care costs continue to increase (in 2007 health care costs had risen to 16% of GNP [MedHeadlines, 2008]), employers are providing incentives for participation in wellness and prevention programs. Employees who engage in wellness programs and demonstrate health-related improvements are being offered discounts on health care premiums or prizes such as MP3 players or cash bonuses (Rotenberk, 2007; Szabo, 2008). Wellness programs continue to counter absenteeism, turnover, and workplace stress, in addition to reducing health care costs, factors that, when combined, cost organizations $300 billion dollars a year (Stambor, 2006).

History of Wellness Programs in Schools

Wellness programs in schools began as an outreach of physical education and health education. Both fields have been part of school curriculum for over 125 years; however, they have generally remained separate from each other and from the other curriculum until the 1970s–

1980s. Before the early 1970s, physical education focused on motor skills such as agility, balance, coordination, power, reaction time, and speed. Health curriculum focused on teaching children proper hygiene skills and basic infection control practices, and briefly discussing rudimentary nutritional concepts.

Since the 1980s, school curriculum has moved away from this dichotomy of health education and physical education and has moved toward developing programs that promote healthy lifestyles. Due to the expanding awareness of the benefits of healthy lifestyles, efforts toward wellness education aim to reach children at a young age in order to prevent illnesses later in life. As the new paradigm of health education has emerged, the curriculum has also changed. In 1980, the Health Related Physical Fitness Manual, distributed by the American Alliance for Health, Physical Education, Recreation, and Dance, changed how physical education was defined. Instead of simply focusing on motor skills, the curriculum began to reflect other health-related issues. Flexibility, cardiorespiratory or aerobic endurance, body composition, and muscular strength and endurance became key components in physical education curriculum (Petray & Cortese, 1988). Physical education and health education were then combined to help children understand and appreciate the interconnection of the two. Children began to learn that their health was not affected by just one aspect of their lifestyle, but by a combination of factors. Some schools are teaching health in all subjects, not only in physical and health education classes. For instance, one program teaches children how to calculate their caloric intake in math classes. By incorporating health-related subject matter into many academic subjects, children learn more about the importance of a healthy lifestyle and how pervasively their health impacts their lives.

Expanding wellness programs in schools remains imperative due to recent trends in child and adolescent health. Data from a midcourse review of *Healthy People 2010*, a set of goals and objectives for health established at the national level, indicate that adolescents may be less fit than in previous decades. Data from 2004 indicated a 50% increase in 12- to 19-year-olds who are overweight or obese compared to figures from 1988–1994 and a plateau in the percentage of adolescents who engage in vigorous physical activity (Park, Brindis, Chang, & Irwin, 2008). Lifetime health programs, and a system of accountability for improved health outcomes via the national *Healthy People* program, have been developed in an attempt to counteract this decline in total fitness.

School health programs have demonstrated success in increasing physical activity and improving nutrition, decreasing substance use, decreasing aggression, and decreasing risky sexual behavior (Murray et al., 2007). However, as funding is often directed towards programs that improve academic achievement, school health programs also need to demonstrate their impact on academic outcomes (Murray et al., 2007).

Philosophy of Wellness

As previously detailed, wellness involves the balance of physical, mental, and spiritual aspects of health. It extends beyond the mere concept of prevention and includes enhancing and maintaining optimal health (Saunders, 1988). Illness, within the wellness model, is defined as an imbalance in one's total self (Edlin & Golanty, 1992) rather than a physical ailment. Waters and Hocker (1991) presented a "wellness" continuum to reflect the idea that health is more than just the absence of disease. At one end of the continuum is "disease" with "wellness potential" at the opposite end. "Absence of disease" was placed in the middle of the continuum to indicate that it is only one step in the process of achieving and maintaining wellness. Maximum wellness is considered the process of working toward achieving full individual potential (Waters & Hocker, 1991).

Wellness emphasizes the importance of a comprehensively healthy lifestyle to prevent illness and maintain health. Such a lifestyle requires personal responsibility for one's own health. According to Edlin and Golanty (1992), it is the responsibility of every individual to enhance his or her sense of well-being by seeking self-healing and fostering a lifestyle and feelings that can help prevent disease. Research purports that exposure to prolonged and high levels of stress can suppress the immune system and contribute to illness (Selye, 1993; Watt et al., 1998). Each individual has the ability to amend detrimental lifestyle habits, reduce stress, and adopt positive habits that promote health. Furthermore, a person's responsibility does not end with the decision to be healthy; wellness is an ongoing effort. Wellness is a lifestyle that encourages a harmonious relationship in body, mind, and feelings; it must be maintained throughout a person's entire life (Edlin & Golanty, 1992).

Music therapy is integral to wellness efforts, as music may be used therapeutically to positively impact immunological, neuroendocrine, and psychological functioning (Bittman et al., 2001; Bittman et al., 2005; Hirokawa & Ohira, 2003; Kuhn, 2002). Both active engagement and receptive participation in music offer benefits, though the nature and degree of response vary with the intervention. As will be discussed in more detail below, active engagement in a group-drumming music therapy protocol or in recreational music-making led to improvements in immunological functioning and improved mood states (Bittman et al., 2001; Bittman, Bruhn, Stevens, Westengard, & Umbach, 2003). Listening to relaxation music reversed stress responses, especially when music was paired with verbal suggestions for relaxation, vibrotactile stimulation, or progressive relaxation exercises (Pelletier, 2004). Participating in amateur singing lessons reduced arousal and improved joyful mood states (Grape, Sandgren, Hansson, Ericson, & Theorell, 2003). Thus, a broad range of therapeutic uses of music may result in the achievement of wellness outcomes.

Music therapy is also attuned to the self-responsibility aspect of the wellness philosophy, as certain therapeutic uses of music, such as stress management music listening programs or music-based wellness exercises, can be self-implemented by individuals as a way to promote a healthy lifestyle. The inherent motivation involved in active music making and music listening may also help to increase adherence to other wellness efforts, such as engagement in exercise programs (Wininger & Pargman, 2003). Additionally, music can be used to structure wellness exercises and lend meaning to wellness techniques that might seem trivial by themselves.

Wellness components of social integration, emotional health, and spirituality are also meaningfully addressed through music therapy. The social elements of music making are optimized in wellness music therapy group work, including stress management programs, therapeutic drum circles, and wellness-based music ensembles, among others. Communal engagement in music serves to decrease isolation, improve social support, and strengthen healthy self-identity. Active music making decreases mood disturbance (Bittman et al., 2003) and offers a supportive outlet for emotional expression (Scheve, 2004). As holistic health encompasses spiritual growth and well-being, music may be used to provide access to spiritual resources in order to optimize wellness (Lipe, 2002). The exact use of music for wellness will vary according to participant age, needs, resources, abilities, and preferences. Interest in the use of music for wellness is not limited to music therapists alone. Music educators are also developing theory and practice to expand the use of music learning and participation for wellness and growth of self for all ends of the age spectrum (Roskam & Reuer, 1999).

Philosophy of Wellness Programs for Older Adults

In order for older individuals to retain their independence and to keep a high quality of life, efforts must be made to achieve wellness and maintain maximum levels of functioning. Maintaining optimal independent functioning in the presence or absence of chronic illness is the cornerstone of wellness in older adults. Addressing and implementing the various dimensions of wellness positively impacts holistic health. If the individual functions optimally by being self-responsible for health, achieving health through nutrition, physical exercise, stress management, socialization, safety through environmental sensitivity, and spiritual development, these efforts will result in the longevity of independence and quality of life (Campbell & Kreidler, 1994; Fitch & Slivinske, 1988; Walker, 1991; Walker, 1992).

Due to the rapid pace and current expectations of our modern hi-tech society, older individuals commonly experience unsatisfactory life qualities. Older individuals are left alive, underemployed, untrained in the latest technologies, and commonly separated from family and community (Miller, 1991). Wellness programs can reverse this lethal cycle and instead focus on improving health, connections to society, and quality of life for older individuals.

Psychosocial theories of aging also lend support to the importance of health promotion for older adults. Hamlin's Utility Theory postulates that societies that strive to keep individuals active and useful during the later years of life actually increase life expectancy (Miller, 1991). If older individuals are given opportunities to remain proactive in life activities and in health matters, they may maintain higher levels of health and well-being. Using and expanding energy as well as remaining active and useful are important aspects of Hamlin's Utility Theory that are directly applicable to a wellness model of health in older adults. By remaining involved in their communities and in society at large, older individuals will receive vital social stimulation, physical exercise, continued independence, and a growing sense of self-responsibility. Supplemental social service and health care programs (such as holistic nursing consultations, nutritional advisement, exercise programs, religious groups, and music therapy programs) can assure that older individuals receive support in the remaining areas of wellness.

The philosophy of the use of music therapy in wellness programs for older adults follows directly from the philosophy of wellness itself. Music, because of its potential to influence physical, social, emotional, and cognitive functioning, is a motivating medium through which wellness techniques may be taught and implemented. Theories derived inductively from research with older populations purport that music therapy techniques can (a) increase motivation and compliance with physical exercise, (b) provide opportunities for meaningful interaction with peers and reduce isolation, (c) provide an outlet for emotional expression and therefore can reduce anxiety and stress, and (d) stimulate active cognitive functioning. Since music therapy wellness programming promotes active engagement and may be more captivating than a general wellness discussion group, music therapy has the potential to increase adherence to long-term wellness lifestyle changes. VanWeelden and Whipple (2004) identify the aptness of music therapy to achieve wellness goals and foresee an increased demand for music therapy wellness programs as the geriatric population increases.

Philosophy of Wellness Programs in Corporations

In the workplace, wellness programs were founded or endorsed by corporations to provide opportunities for employees to become aware of the importance of good health (Benzold, Carlson, & Peck, 1986; Glasgow & Terborg, 1988). Self-awareness and self-responsibility for health guide individuals to make positive changes in their behaviors and lifestyle in order to enhance their overall health (Anspaugh et al., 1995; Benzold et al., 1986). Practicing healthy behaviors within an overall healthy lifestyle prevents or lessens the impact of diseases, disabilities, and injuries (Pender, Walker, Sechrist, & Frank-Stromborg, 1990). Because of these wellness efforts, employees enhance their health and make fewer medical claims, maintain productivity levels, reduce absenteeism, and report increased job satisfaction (Parks & Steelman, 2008). Ultimately, wellness efforts result in an overall increase in profit for companies that use such programs because they lead to reduction in health care costs and may reduce turnover.

Despite the demonstrated economic and quality of life benefits of corporate wellness programs, employers still struggle to entice employees to commence and maintain wellness efforts and make lasting lifestyle changes. Successful use of music therapy in corporate wellness settings hinges on the power of music to motivate, energize, and reinforce individuals who are attempting to make healthy lifestyle changes. The active music-making process may provide motivation for meaningful engagement and improve adherence to wellness programming. Music therapy wellness programs may be scheduled for short periods during the course of the workday to facilitate employee participation without impacting leisure time outside of work. Programs for music listening during exercise may promote exercise enjoyment and increase adherence to physical fitness (Wininger & Pargman, 2003).

In addition to improving adherence to lifestyle changes, music therapy in the work setting decreases the impact of stress on immune functioning and provides an emotional outlet and social support to improve mood states and decrease burnout (Bittman et al., 2005; Bittman et al., 2003; Wachi et al., 2007). The use of music therapy in corporate settings is also cost-effective, as positive outcomes have been consistently demonstrated after six sessions of a recreational music-making protocol (Bittman et al., 2003), or in as little as a single session of group drumming music therapy (Bittman et al., 2001).

Philosophy of Wellness Programs in Schools

Developing wellness programs in schools is crucial as children are at the ideal age to learn the skills and mindset for a wellness-based lifestyle. If wellness habits are adopted in childhood, individuals will reap benefits throughout the lifespan. Young children are frequently curious about who they are and how their bodies develop and grow and are eager to find ways to relate to the world about them (Koss & Ketcham, 1980). This inquisitive stage is the perfect time to teach children the components of a healthy lifestyle. Early lessons and practice in wellness behaviors will prevent many unhealthy habits from forming.

According to Koss and Ketcham (1980), wellness programs in schools need to counteract the social norms of today's "illness culture." The average American child watches television 25 hours per week, rides a school bus, consumes high-fat foods, and lacks motivation to exercise regularly (Sweetgall & Neeves, 1987). Children should be made aware of the long-term impact their health-related decisions have on their lives and the importance of maintaining a healthy lifestyle in order to avoid health problems later in life.

Music therapy can be integrated into school wellness programs to achieve wellness outcomes. Music provides hands-on experiences, which are essential in instructing young children. Through these experiences, music can motivate, stimulate, and facilitate children's learning. A supportive environment can be established by adding familiar music, either through active music making or by prerecorded music used as a background for an activity. Music may be used to gain and prolong attention, structure the activity, or serve as a cue. Using music as a mnemonic device may improve recall and enhance learning (Thaut, Peterson, & McIntosh, 2005). By using song lyrics as information carriers, children can retain learned wellness information longer; therefore, they will be more likely to implement these health-based concepts into their lifestyles. Music therapy used in a classroom setting can also teach children the value of positive social interaction, communication, and cooperation. Implementing music in classroom wellness activities also offers opportunities to involve students in the planning process of their wellness program. By learning how to select appropriate music to facilitate wellness techniques, children are able to structure and support their own personal wellness programs.

Description of Wellness Programs

Wellness programming offers instruction and support to participants as they go through the steps of assessing their current lifestyles, formulating goals and objectives, planning strategies to work toward these goals, and implementing lifestyle changes. Evaluation of the outcomes of these lifestyle changes is important for the continual adjustment of wellness efforts. Since wellness programs stress the lifelong process of maintaining health, these steps will be continually repeated and adjusted as participants strive for their optimal holistic health.

Effective wellness programs include a variety of the previously mentioned components of holistic health. Specific program components will vary according to the needs, abilities, and life circumstances of the participants. Most components of wellness are valuable to any population, but varying levels of emphasis will be placed on the various components depending on the characteristics of the participants.

Description of Wellness Programs for Older Adults

Wellness programs for older individuals emphasize components common to most general wellness programs along with personal safety, socialization, intellectual stimulation, and screening for depression or other mental health issues. Promoting personal safety by engaging in health-protecting behaviors, such as adapting home environments to prevent falls and fires, is important for this age group. Wellness programs for older individuals may also offer intellectual stimulation (Crowley, 1992) to promote maintenance of cognitive functioning. Interpersonal support may include opportunities for socialization or community involvement. Periodic visits with health care personnel are important in order to monitor health conditions and also increase the chance of early diagnosis of mental health problems (Wilson et al., 1989).

Wellness programs for older adults have demonstrated promising results. Research indicates that older adults are quite interested in health promotion (Viverais-Dresler, Bakker, & Vance, 1995; White & Nezey, 1996); that they view "being well" as being independent and free from pain (Campbell & Kreidler, 1994); that older adults who are actively working, volunteering or otherwise, or who are interacting with their communities are generally more positive about their well-being (Campbell & Kreidler, 1994; Crowley, 1992); and, most importantly, that older individuals are willing to make lifestyle changes in order to achieve wellness (Campbell & Kreidler, 1994, Viverais-Dresler et al., 1995). Wellness programs have also promoted physical wellness of older adults (Crowley, 1992; White & Nezey, 1996), and increased educational and social support outcomes (Ruffing-Rahal, 1993). Nevertheless, many older adults perceive their health status as being out of their control (Campbell & Kreidler, 1994). They view their physicians as authority figures and tend to never second-guess a physician's judgment (Campbell & Kreidler, 1994). Older adults may need to be convinced of their own strong potential to positively influence their health in order to increase the potency of wellness programs.

Music therapy is currently used in a variety of ways to address the following dimensions of wellness in older adults: physical fitness, interpersonal support, intellectual stimulation, stress management, self-actualization, and spiritual development. These goal areas are addressed through a variety of wellness music therapy interventions including senior adult choirs, intergenerational choirs, music-supported movement programs, keyboard lessons paired with music therapy wellness exercises, intergenerational music skills development groups, and therapeutic drumming (Clair, 1996; Clair, in press; Hamburg & Clair, in press; Koga, 2005; Roskam & Reuer, 1999; VanWeelden & Whipple, 2004).

Music can increase enjoyment of exercise, enhance motivation, and help structure movement, leading to improved commitment to exercise for older adults (Clair, 1996). Tempo is an important quality associated with music enjoyment during exercise (Wininger & Pargman, 2003) and should be matched to the purpose of the exercise and the participant's functional ability. Other aspects of rhythm may help cue movement, influencing movement duration, speed, and range of motion (Hamburg & Clair, 2003b). A series of studies has examined the impact of music specifically composed to reflect the structure of movements during an exercise program for older adults. Weekly participation in a wellness-based movement and music program led to increases in one-foot stance balance, gait speed, and functional reach after five sessions (Hamburg & Clair, 2003b). These positive results were supported in a larger study, which demonstrated improved measures of balance and gait characteristics after 5 weeks of the music and movement protocol (Hamburg & Clair, 2003a). Such programs have the potential to promote gains in physical functioning, maintain independence, and improve quality of life for older adults (Hamburg & Clair, 2003b).

Older adults who engage in music making as part of a group receive valuable social support and may develop a healthy sense of belonging. Although depressive disorders are not highly prevalent among older adults, they pose serious consequences to health and levels of functioning, as a higher suicide rate is reported for this group than any other (Chapman & Perry, 2008). Group music engagement can help build relationships between older adults with similar interests, overcoming a tendency toward isolation brought on by limited mobility, physical frailty, and mental incapacity (Hays, Bright, & Minichiello, 2002). Music facilitates this social bridging which, when combined with the exercise and emotive aspects inherent in active music making, may help improve mood and alleviate depression among older participants.

By learning to self-implement music therapy wellness techniques, older individuals also improve their personal responsibility for health. Preferred stimulative or sedative music may be used at certain times of the day to promote activity or relaxation and to modulate mood in a desired direction. Hays et al. (2002) emphasized music's capacity to positively affect mood and mental states in older adults and stated that music may provide an opportunity for emotional expression and catharsis. Music therapy also promotes the processes of personal growth and intellectual stimulation that combine to maintain intellectual functioning in older adults. Development or relearning of music skills requires active cognition and recall, challenges fine motor skills, and can promote positive self-esteem and a sense of achievement.

Reducing stress is important to overall health since prolonged stress depresses immune functioning. Music may be paired with relaxation techniques to facilitate stress management. Music should be sedative and should match the pace of the relaxation exercise, as well as be tailored to the listener's preferences. Relaxation techniques used in music therapy wellness programs may include deep breathing exercises, suggestions for relaxation, progressive muscle relaxation, slow stretching movements, or music and imagery techniques. Pilot study results from a music therapy wellness program by Clair (1998) supported the use of music therapy to reduce the negative effects of anxiety and stress on older adults.

Clair (1998) developed an active music-making wellness program for healthy older individuals that incorporates the use of piano keyboards. These various self-implemented wellness techniques include various breathing exercises, muscle relaxation exercises, cognitive strategies to encourage positive thinking and increase confidence, techniques for using music to stimulate or sedate behavior, and strategies for using music to influence mood. A multidisciplinary team of researchers, operating within the "Music Making and Wellness Project," investigated the use of such a program of weekly keyboard lessons paired with music therapy wellness activities over the course of a 5-year span. Decreases in anxiety, depression, and perception of loneliness were reported for the 50 older adults in the experimental group (Bruhn & Clair, 1999; Koga, 2005). The study also identified a 90% increase in levels of human growth hormone, of which higher levels have been linked to increased energy and sexual function, and to decreased occurrence of illnesses related to aging (Koga, 2005). Research in the field of music therapy, wellness, and gerontology is expanding, and findings from such research demonstrate the far-reaching benefits of a music-based wellness approach for older adults.

Description of Wellness Programs in Corporations

The U.S. government has recently begun to publicly recognize the importance of health promotion in the workplace. The governmental study *Healthy People 2000* (Public Health Service, 1990) had a national objective of increasing employee health promotion activities in at least 85% of workplaces with 50 or more employees. In the last three decades, corporate America has recognized the potential of wellness programs, with an estimated 90% of American businesses providing health promotion activities to their employees (Aldana et al., 2005). Numerous health promotion activities are used in the workplace. Programs vary from company to company due to different needs, interests, and support of employers and employees, and due to the size and scope of the health promotion intervention (Levy, 1986; Risner & Fowler, 1995). Physical fitness, nutrition, stress management, counseling, weight control, high blood pressure treatment, lifestyle consultation, discussion groups, health screening, health education, on-site physical examinations, on-site physical therapy, safety awareness education, health risk appraisal, hypertension control, leisure activities, and smoking and alcohol cessation programs are examples of corporate wellness interventions.

Among the various wellness components, stress management has been the most attractive for employers (Ivancevich, Matteson, Freedman, & Phillips, 1990). Prolonged stress is correlated with a variety of health problems such as coronary heart disease, cancer, diabetes, and depression, and it results in nearly one million U.S. workers missing work each day (Jacobson et al., 1996). Stress not only provokes disease and injury, but it can cause other problems in the workplace such as reduced productivity, disloyalty, job dissatisfaction, poor decision making, high turnover, increased error, and damage and waste. A recent meta-analysis of occupational stress management programs found that cognitive-behavioral interventions were the most effective methods for managing stress, though relaxation and meditation techniques were more frequently offered in such programs (Richardson & Rothstein, 2008).

Fitness and exercise programs have also been popular parts of corporate wellness programs. Lack of daily physical exercise has been recognized as a contributing factor to many chronic diseases such as coronary artery disease, cancer, and work-related injuries (Anspaugh et al., 1995). Other benefits of exercise and fitness include reducing stress, boosting energy, lowering cholesterol levels and high blood pressure, increasing productivity, and reducing the turnover rate (Shephard, 1996).

Recreational activities are also used in corporate wellness programs. SAS Institute, Inc. and Sentry provide programs such as basketball, volleyball, softball, billiards, karate, and social dance. Ragheb (1993) found a strong relationship between leisure satisfaction and perceived wellness. Participation in reading and social activities had an especially strong relationship to the perceived wellness of employees. The author suggested that companies make more of an effort to provide services such as company libraries and recreational facilities where employees can engage in social activities.

There is a documented history, dating back to the 19th century, of using recorded music in factories and work settings to boost morale and productivity. Tempo and rhythms of the music were matched to rhythms of the work to maintain production speeds (le Roux, 2005). Occasionally song lyrics were used to raise public awareness of poor working conditions, with an aim of improving workers' long-term health. More recently, recorded music has been piped into stairwells to increase stair use (Boutelle, Jeffery, Murray, & Schmitz, 2001). Today, new uses of music, primarily through active music making, are positively impacting the health and well-being of working adults.

The past decade has evidenced an increase in research and clinical programs utilizing music therapy and therapeutic uses of music to promote wellness outcomes in work settings. Representatives from the music industry are pairing with music therapists and researchers to promote the use of active music making for health and wellness. The Remo, Inc. HealthRHYTHMS division is one example of this trend. The HealthRHYTHMS division "develops and provides materials, programs, training and the latest research supporting the use of drumming as an effective means for promoting and maintaining health and well-being" (Remo, Inc., 2008). This collaboration has led to the development and research testing of therapeutic group drumming protocols.

Bittman et al. (2001) described a single-session group drumming music therapy protocol incorporating a warm-up of a light-hearted rhythmic challenge, rhythmic naming, group drumming, and a guided imagery experience in which participants drummed in variation with the spoken imagery. This single 1-hour session was immunoenhancing, modulating specific neuroendocrine and neuroimmune parameters in a direction opposite of the classic stress response for the healthy adult participants (Bittman et al., 2001). Therapeutic drumming protocols were also effectively used with long-term care workers and first-year associate degree nursing students. Participation in a six-session Recreational Music-making (RMM) protocol reduced multiple dimensions of burnout and improved mood states in both long-term care workers and in first-year associate degree nursing students (Bittman et al., 2003; Bittman et al., 2004). This RMM protocol utilized Group Empowerment Drumming, coupled with a series of wellness exercises using keyboards (Bittman et al., 2003). Both studies estimated substantial cost savings related to potentially reducing employee turnover by using RMM to reduce multiple parameters associated with burnout.

Participation in a single session of the Recreational Music-making protocol following a stress-induction period resulted in a greater reversal of stress response, at the level of genomic expression, than the resting control group (Bittman et al., 2005). Healthy male corporate employees participated in a single session of the RMM protocol and demonstrated improved mood and modulated levels of natural killer cell activity toward the normal range, which equates with reversal of stress response (Wachi et al., 2007). Apart from therapeutic drumming, other active uses of music have proven beneficial to healthy adults. Kuhn (2002) found active music participation (singing and playing small percussive instruments) produced a greater effect on the immune system as measured by Salivary Immunoglobulin A (SIgA) than passive listening to live music, though both were more beneficial than a nonmusic control group.

Passive therapeutic uses of music have also demonstrated beneficial effects in healthy individuals. Pelletier (2004) conducted a meta-analysis of the use of pre-recorded music and music-assisted relaxation techniques and found a large effect size, suggesting that both significantly decreased arousal due to stress. Subjects under the age of 18 years showed greater benefit that those who were older, and effect sizes were greatest for adolescents in their third trimester preparing for labor and in studies with artificially induced stress. Verbal suggestion with music, music with vibrotactile stimulation, and music-assisted progressive relaxation were more effective for reducing stress than music listening alone (Pelletier, 2004). Results of this meta-analysis suggest that music selected on the basis of research elicited better stress reduction than music selected by the subject, and that participants with prior musical experience demonstrated greater stress reduction than those without.

Several studies not included in the above meta-analysis have demonstrated additional wellness-related benefits of pre-recorded music. The Bonny Method of Guided Imagery and Music (GIM) was implemented with healthy adults and, after six biweekly sessions, resulted in decreased depression, fatigue, and total mood disturbance, as well as reduced cortisol levels by 6-week follow-up (McKinney, Antoni, Kumar, Tims, & McCabe, 1997). Relaxation music reduced anxiety from experimentally induced stress in healthy adults (Knight & Rickard, 2001;

Walworth, 2003) and prevented stress-induced changes in physiological measures (Knight & Rickard, 2001). Walworth (2003) demonstrated that using songs from a listener-preferred genre or artist was as effective at reducing anxiety as using a specific listener-preferred song. Listening to a relaxing classical music selection resulted in more psychological relaxation and less stress than listening to a New Age relaxation selection or reading preferred magazines (Smith & Joyce, 2004). Stimulative and sedative music has varying effects on immunity, neuroendocrine responses, and psychological measures in healthy subjects. Hirokawa and Ohira (2003) found that stimulative music decreased depression, increased liveliness and norepinephrine level (indicating excitement of the sympathetic nervous system), and promoted recovery of natural killer cell activity after an induced stressor. Alternatively, sedative music facilitated relaxation, decreased physiological arousal, and increased sense of well-being, but it was also correlated with suppressed indicators of immune function.

In his review of the use of music listening to promote relaxation and wellness, Krout (2006) mentioned three levels at which music may be used for wellness. Music for wellness may be a health treatment provided by a qualified music therapist, it may consist of wellness techniques established by a music therapist for a client's independent implementation, or it may include the appropriate use of music by other allied health professionals to promote wellness benefits. Krout provided a rationale for the efficacy of a personalized music listening and relaxation program to promote wellness and gave suggestions for dealing with logistics related to the implementation of such a technique. Wolfe, O'Connell, and Waldon (2002) noted that the majority of nonmusicians in their study of relaxation music preferences reported using music "daily" or "several times per week" while relaxing. This propensity to use music while relaxing, when coupled with the research regarding positive outcomes from music listening, indicates that music listening programs may be an important area of clinical practice in wellness music therapy. Given increasing knowledge of the effect of music listening on arousal, immune functioning, and mood states, as well as implications from research regarding music preference and qualities of the music chosen and its use, music therapists may create clinically effective listening programs for their clients to achieve wellness outcomes.

Therapeutic drumming protocols and music listening for stress management are well-supported by research and should be incorporated into clinical wellness music therapy efforts in corporate settings. The development and use of music-assisted stress management programs incorporating cognitive-behavioral interventions is also indicated by the literature. Other evidence-based approaches incorporating GIM, singing, or music to structure exercise show promise, and future research could help to strengthen the use of these approaches for wellness in corporate settings.

Description of Wellness Programs in Schools

The curriculum content of wellness programs in schools is broad and covers many areas. In 1984, the National Professional School Health Education Organization identified 10 areas of health instruction. Half of these areas included different types of health, including community health, consumer health, environmental health, nutritional health, and personal health. Family life, growth and development, prevention and control of diseases and disorders, safety and accident prevention, and substance use and abuse made up the other 5 areas (Petray & Cortese,

1988). Since this list was published, other areas have been identified as important aspects of a comprehensive wellness education program. Fitness, lifestyle choices, personal responsibility, emotional health, and stress management are also commonly included in wellness programs. Other areas that are typically covered are avoiding risky behaviors; enjoying life; genetics; healthy communication; the influence of peers, family, community, and media on our decisions; and spiritual awareness.

Although music has not yet been systematically integrated into school wellness programs, it carries good potential for increasing the overall effectiveness of wellness programs. To date, most occurrences of music in wellness programs have been in the form of instructional songs used to help younger children remember health information. For instance, one program included a song to the tune "If You're Happy and You Know It." The lyrics were replaced with directives that instructed children to use tissues when they sneezed and to cover their mouths when they coughed. Other wellness programs have included songs that remind children how to brush their teeth properly or that teach children what foods they should eat (Bromberg et al., 1995).

School programs have also included music in stress management instruction. Giles, Cogan, and Cox (1991) studied the use of music to alter negative moods of children and prepare them for learning. This study developed out of the observed increase in behavior disorders resulting from marked emotional stress. The researchers used music and art as means to deal with stress, leading to improved emotional health and an improved learning environment. Other stress management techniques involving music can also be taught to children. Music can be used to structure breathing exercises as well as techniques such as progressive muscle relaxation.

Culturally relevant music may be used as a tool to promote health maintenance in adolescents and young adults. Stephens, Braithwaite, and Taylor (1998) created a clinical model that uses current hip-hop music and lyric analysis to promote HIV/AIDS prevention among young African American adolescents. The authors contended that the use of culturally relevant music is clinically effective, as song messages are created and delivered by peers and thus gain the attention of participants, music promotes a proactive positive response and motivates participants, and music promotes self-expression. The familiar hip-hop songs are used to identify high-risk behaviors, to facilitate role-play based on song content, and to promote development of healthy problem-solving skills. The authors recommended that future use and empirical testing of this model might also encompass other health promotion activities such as violence reduction and substance abuse prevention (Stephens et al., 1998).

Other therapeutic uses of music for wellness in the school setting reflect generalization of evidence-based practice from adult populations. Music can be used to motivate participation in the physical fitness component of the wellness program. Music therapists can teach children how to use music to structure physical fitness activities as they learn how to develop their own fitness programs. Encouraging children to choose their own music may help motivate them to develop their own daily exercise programs and self-implement these programs.

In a classroom setting, music therapy wellness programs would most likely take place in groups. In music ensembles, issues such as personal responsibility, healthy communication, influence of peers, and positive interactions are addressed. Participation in active music making may allow children an outlet for emotional expression, potentially leading to more stability of mood. A music therapist may use the group setting and interpersonal dynamics to teach and practice healthy conflict resolution and anger management skills. Music therapy sessions can also provide children with a chance to develop positive leisure skills. Participating in these productive hobbies could prevent children from choosing high-risk behaviors as they grow older or prevent them from falling into sedentary lifestyles. Musical hobbies can also provide an emotional outlet and a refreshing break from the regular routine of schoolwork. Developing musical skills can also allow children to become actively involved in their communities.

Considerations and Conclusions

The wellness movement is gaining popularity in various sectors of our society, though obstacles to its widespread acceptance remain. Resistance to the development of the wellness movement in the field of health care stems from concerns over the immediacy of wellness benefits, lack of reimbursement for physician-provided wellness services (Goldman, Adamson, Raymond, & Schore, 1989), restrictions of the present fee-for-service structure, lack of health care worker training in implementing wellness programs, and reluctance to alter the traditional paradigm of health care. Despite the recent growth of corporate wellness programs, employers are frequently forced to provide incentives to encourage and maintain employee participation (Rotenberk, 2007). Small businesses have trouble supporting comprehensive wellness programs. Thus, many employees may not have access to wellness programs. Also, corporate health promotion programs may focus on reduction of physical and mental problems to the detriment of addressing higher states of well-being such as creativity and group cohesion (Stokols et al., 1996). Resistance in school settings stems from a reluctance to change well-ingrained educational traditions; lack of resources, time, and effort to create comprehensive wellness programs; and the reality that funding is frequently limited to programs that clearly improve academic achievement. Even if all of these obstacles are conquered, developing individual self-reliance and self-responsibility for health will remain a challenge.

Creating and listening to music offer benefits that impact nearly every domain of wellness. These benefits are valid and relevant for all age groups. Evidence from recent research in the field helps identify areas for evidenced-based clinical practice in wellness music therapy and gives direction for future development. Music therapists are encouraged to serve as pioneers in this emergent area of clinical practice, developing and expanding upon approaches that are firmly founded in research and theory.

Health care professionals, businesses, and the population at large are beginning to recognize the benefits of a holistic wellness approach to health care. They also comprehend the connection between the body, mind, and spirit and the influences each has on the other. As increasing numbers of people begin to take responsibility for their own health, there will be increasing demand for enjoyable approaches of developing healthier lifestyles and maintaining health. Music therapy is a versatile wellness intervention that can be adapted and adjusted to facilitate and maintain a lifestyle of wellness for individuals across the life span.

References

Aldana, S. G., Merrill, R. M., Price, K., Hardy, A., & Hager, R. (2005). Financial impact of a comprehensive multisite workplace health promotion program. *Preventive Medicine, 4*, 31–137.

American Music Therapy Association (AMTA). (2005). *AMTA Standards of Clinical Practice*. Silver Spring, MD: Author.

Anspaugh, D. J., Hunter, S., & Mosley, J. (1995). The economic impact of corporate wellness programs: Past and future considerations. *AAOHN Journal, 43*(4), 203–210.

Benson, E. R., & McDevitt, J. Q. (1989). Home care and the older adult: Illness care versus wellness care. *Holistic Nursing Practice, 3*(2), 30–38.

Benzold, C., Carlson, R. J., & Peck, J. C. (1986). *The future of work and health*. Dover, MA: Auburn House.

Bittman, B., Berk, L., Shannon, M., Sharaf, M., Westengard, J., Guegler, K. J., & Ruff, D. W. (2005). Recreational music-making modulates the human stress response: A preliminary individualized gene expression strategy. *Medical Science Monitor, 11*(2), BR31–BR40.

Bittman, B., Berk, L. S., Felten, D. L., Westengard, J., Simonton, O. C., Pappas, J., et al. (2001). Composite effects of group drumming music therapy on modulation of neuroendocrine-immune parameters in normal subjects. *Alternative Therapies in Health and Medicine, 7*(1), 38–47.

Bittman, B., Bruhn, K. T., Stevens, C., Westengard, J., & Umbach, P. O. (2003). Recreational music-making: A cost-effective group interdisciplinary strategy for reducing burnout and improving mood states in long-term care workers. *Advances in Mind-Body Medicine, 19*(3/4), 4–15.

Bittman, B. B., Snyder, C., Bruhn, K. T., Liebfreid, F., Stevens, C. K., Westengard, J., & Umbach, P. O. (2004). Recreational music-making: An integrative group intervention for reducing burnout and improving mood states in first year associate degree nursing students: Insights and economic impact. *International Journal of Nursing Education Scholarship, 1*(1), Article 12.

Boutelle, K. N., Jeffery, R. W., Murray, D. M., & Schmitz, M. K. (2001). Using signs, artwork, and music to promote stair use in a public building. *American Journal of Public Health, 91*(12), 2004–2006.

Bromberg, B., Chiu, C., Dollman, K., Hansen, L., Kim, C. Y., Lessen, B., et al. (1995). *Health wellness and Hospital Learning Center*. Buffalo, NY: Early Childhood Research Center.

Bruhn, K. T., & Clair, A. A. (1999, July). *Active music making and wellness*. Remo HealthRHYTHMS. Retrieved May 8, 2008, from http://www.remo.com/portal/pages/health_rhythms/library_article1.html

Bulaclac, M. C. (1996). A work site wellness program. *Nursing Management, 27*(12), 19–22.

Campbell, J., & Kreidler, M. (1994). Older adults' perceptions about wellness. *Journal of Holistic Nursing, 12*, 437–447.

Chapman, D. P., & Perry, G. S. (2008). Depression as a major component of public health for older adults. *Preventing Chronic Disease: Public Health Research, Practice, and Policy, 5*(1), 1–9.

Chenoweth, D. (1991). *Planning health promotion at the worksite*. Dubuque, IA: Brown & Benchmark.

Clair, A. A. (1996). *Therapeutic uses of music with older adults*. Baltimore: Health Professions Press.

Clair, A. A. (1998). *Active music making and wellness applications*. Unpublished manuscript, University of Kansas, Lawrence.

Clair, A. A., & Memmott, J. (2008). *Therapeutic uses of music with older adults*. Silver Spring, MD: American Music Therapy Association.

Crowley, M., Sr. (1992). Living longer and better than expected. *Health Progress, 73*(10), 38–41.

Dunn, G. H. (1959). What high-level wellness means. *Canadian Journal of Public Health, 50*, 447–457.

Ebersole, P., & Hess, P. (1981). *Toward healthy aging: Human needs and nursing response*. St. Louis, MO: C. V. Mosby.

Edlin, G., & Golanty, E. (1992). *Health and wellness: A holistic approach*. Boston: Jones & Bartlett.

Fitch, V. L., & Slivinske, L. R. (1988). Maximizing effects of wellness programs for the elderly. *Health & Social Work, 13*(1), 61–67.

Giles, M. M., Cogan, D., & Cox, C. (1991). A music and art program to promote emotional health in elementary school children. *Journal of Music Therapy, 28*, 135–148.

Glasgow, R. E., & Terborg, J. R. (1988). Occupational health promotion programs to reduce cardiovascular risk. *Journal of Consulting and Clinical Psychology, 56*(3), 365–373.

Goldman, R. L., Adamson, T. E., Raymond, G. L., & Schore, J. E. (1989). It is time to move from health maintenance to health promotion. *Journal of Hospital Marketing, 3*, 105–119.

Goldsmith, M. F. (1986). Worksite wellness programs: Latest wrinkle to smooth health care costs. *Journal of the American Medical Association, 256*(9), 1089–1095.

Grape, C., Sandgren, M., Hansson, L.-O., Ericson, M., & Theorell, T. (2003). Does singing promote well-being?: An empirical study of professional and amateur singers during a singing lesson. *Integrative Physiological & Behavioral Science, 38*(1), 65–74.

Gutt, C. A. (1996). Health and wellness in the community. In J. M. Cookfair (Ed.), *Nursing care in the community* (2nd ed., pp. 143–174). St. Louis, MO: Mosby.

Hamburg, J., & Clair, A. A. (2003a). The effects of a Laban-based movement program with music on measures of balance and gait in older adults. *Activities, Adaptations, & Aging, 28*, 17–33.

Hamburg, J., & Clair, A. A. (2003b). The effects of a movement with music program on measures of balance and gait speed in healthy older adults. *Journal of Music Therapy, 40*(3), 212–227.

Hamburg, J., & Clair, A. A. (in press). The effects of a Laban/Bartenieff-based movement program with music on physical function measures in older adults. *Music Therapy Perspectives*.

Hays, T., Bright, R., & Minichiello, V. (2002). The contribution of music to positive aging: A review. *Journal of Aging and Identity, 7*(3), 165–175.

Hirokawa, E., & Ohira, H. (2003). The effects of music listening after a stressful task on immune functions, neuroendocrine responses, and emotional states in college students. *Journal of Music Therapy, 40*(3), 189–211.

Ivancevich, J. M., Matteson, M. T., Freedman, S. M., & Phillips, J. S. (1990). Worksite stress management interventions. *American Psychologist, 45*(2), 252–261.

Jacobson, B. H., Aldana, S. G., Goetzel, R. Z., Vardell, K. D., Adams, T. B., & Pietras, R. J. (1996). The relationship between perceived stress and self-reported illness-related absenteeism. *American Journal of Health Promotion, 11*(1), 54–61.

Knight, W. E., & Rickard, N. S. (2001). Relaxing music prevents stress-induced increases in subjective anxiety, systolic blood pressure, and heart rate in healthy males and females. *Journal of Music Therapy, 38*(4), 254–272.

Koga, M. (2005, October/November). The Music Making and Wellness Project. *American Music Teacher*.

Koss, L., & Ketcham, M. (1980). *Building wellness lifestyles: Counselor's manual*. Morristown, NJ: Human Resources Institute.

Krout, R. E. (2006). Music listening to facilitate relaxation and promote wellness: Integrated aspects of our neurophysiological responses to music. *The Arts in Psychotherapy, 34*, 134–141.

Kuhn, D. (2002). The effects of active and passive participation in musical activity on the immune system as measured by salivary immunoglobulin A (SIgA). *Journal of Music Therapy, 39*(1), 30–39.

le Roux, G. M. (2005). "Whistle while you work": A historical account of some associations among music, work, and health. *American Journal of Public Health, 95*(7), 1106–1109.

Levy, S. R. (1986). Work site health promotion. *Family and Community Health, 9*(3), 51–62.

Lipe, A. W. (2002). Beyond therapy: Music, spirituality, and health in human experience: A review of literature. *Journal of Music Therapy, 39*(3), 209–240.

McKinney, C. H., Antoni, M. H., Kumar, M., Tims, F. C., & McCabe, P. M. (1997). Effects of guided imagery and music (GIM) therapy on mood and cortisol in healthy adults. *Health Psychology, 16*(4), 390–400.

MedHeadlines. (2008, February). *Health care 16.3% of GDP and climbing.* Retrieved June 2, 2008, from, http://medheadlines.com/2008/02/26/health-care-163-of-gdp-and-climbing/

Miller, M. P. (1991). Factors promoting wellness in the aged person: An ethnographic study. *Advances in Nursing Science, 13*(4), 38–51.

Murray, N. G., Low, B. J., Hollis, C., Cross, A. W., & Davis, S. M. (2007). Coordinated school health programs and academic achievement: A systematic review of the literature. *Journal of School Health, 77*(9), 589–600.

Park, M. J., Brindis, C. D., Chang, F., & Irwin, C. E. (2008). A midcourse review of the healthy people 2010: 21 critical health objectives for adolescents and young adults. *Journal of Adolescent Health, 42*, 328–334.

Parks, K. M., & Steelman, L. A. (2008). Organizational wellness programs: A meta-analysis. *Journal of Occupational Health Psychology, 13*(1), 58–68.

Pelletier, C. L. (2004). The effect of music on decreasing arousal due to stress: A meta-analysis. *Journal of Music Therapy, 41*(3), 192–214.

Pender, N. J., Walker, S. N., Sechrist, K. R., & Frank-Stromborg, M. (1990). Predicting health-promoting lifestyle in the workplace. *Nursing Research, 39*(6), 326–332.

Petray, C. K., & Cortese, P. A. (1988). Physical fitness: A vital component of the school health education curriculum. *Health Education, 19*(5), 4–7.

Public Health Service. (1990). *Healthy People 2000: National health promotion and disease prevention objectives.* Washington, DC: U.S. Government Printing Office.

Ragheb, M. G. (1993). Leisure and perceived wellness: A field investigation. *Leisure Sciences, 15*, 13–24.

Remo, Inc. (2008). *Remo® HealthRHYTHMS: Welcome to HealthRHYTHMS.* Retrieved June 9, 2008, from http://www.remo.com/portal/pages/health_rhythms/index.html

Richardson, K. M., & Rothstein, H. R. (2008). Effects of occupational stress management intervention programs: A meta-analysis. *Journal of Occupational Health Psychology, 13*(1), 69–93.

Risner, P. B., & Fowler, B. A. (1995). Health promotion services and evaluation in the workplace: Pragmatic issues. *AAOHN Journal, 43*(1), 12–16.

Roskam, K., & Reuer, B. (1999). A music therapy wellness model for illness prevention. In C. Dileo (Ed.), *Music therapy and medicine: Theoretical and clinical applications* (pp. 139–147). Silver Spring, MD: American Music Therapy Association.

Rotenberk, L. (2007). Wellness programs gain popularity, take on new approaches. *Hospitals & Health Networks, 81*(8), 30.

Ruffing-Rahal, M. A. (1993). An ecological model of group well-being: Implications for health promotion with older women. *Health Care for Women International, 14,* 447–456.

Saunders, R. P. (1988). What is health promotion? *Health Education, 19*(5), 14–18.

Scheve, A. (2004). Music therapy, wellness, and stress reduction. *Advances in Experimental Medicine and Biology, 546,* 253–263.

Selye, H. (1993). History of the stress concept. In L. Goldberger & S. Breznitz (Eds.), *Handbook of stress: Theoretical and clinical aspects* (2nd ed., pp. 7–20). New York: Free Press.

Shephard, R. J. (1996). Financial aspects of employee fitness programs. In J. Kerr, A. Griffiths, & T. Cox (Eds.), *Workplace health: Employee fitness and exercise* (pp. 29–54). London: Taylor & Francis.

Smith, J. C., & Joyce, C. A. (2004). Mozart versus New Age music: Relaxation states, stress, and ABC relaxation theory. *Journal of Music Therapy, 41*(3), 215–224.

Stambor, Z. (2006, March). Employees: A company's best asset. *Monitor on Psychology, 37,* 28–30.

Stephens, T., Braithwaite, R. L., & Taylor, S. E. (1998). Model for using hip-hop music for small group HIV/AIDS prevention counseling with African American adolescents and young adults. *Patient Education and Counseling, 35,* 127–137.

Stokols, D. S., Pelletier, K. R., & Fielding, J. E. (1996). The ecology of work and health: Research and policy directions for the promotion of employee health. *Health Education Quarterly, 23*(2), 137–158.

Sweetgall, R., & Neeves, R. (1987). *The Walking Wellness teacher's guide: A resource book for elementary and middle school teachers.* Newark, DE: Creative Walking.

Szabo, J. (2008). Wellness and prevention. Taking wellness efforts to employers' doors. *Hospitals and Health Networks, 82*(1), 14.

Thaut, M. H., Peterson, D. A., & McIntosh, G. C. (2005). Temporal entrainment of cognitive functions: Musical mnemonics induce brain plasticity and oscillatory synchrony in neural networks underlying memory. *Annals of the New York Academy of Sciences, 1060,* 243–254.

Travis, J. (1977). *Wellness workbook: A guide to higher level wellness.* Mill Valley, CA: Wellness Resource Center.

VanWeelden, K., & Whipple, J. (2004). Effect of field experiences on music therapy students' perceptions of choral music for geriatric wellness programs. *Journal of Music Therapy, 41*(4), 340–352.

Viverais-Dresler, G. A., Bakker, D. A., & Vance, R. J. (1995). Elderly clients' perceptions: Individual health counseling and group sessions. *Canadian Journal of Public Health, 86,* 234–237.

Wachi, M., Koyama, M., Utsuyama, M., Bittman, B. B., Kitagawa, M., & Hirokawa, K. (2007). Recreational music-making modulates natural killer cell activity, cytokines, and mood states in corporate employees. *Medical Science Monitor, 13*(2), CR57–CR70.

Walker, S. N. (1991). Wellness and aging. In E. M. Baines (Ed.), *Perspectives on gerontological nursing* (pp. 41–58). Newbury Park, CA: Sage.

Walker, S. N. (1992). Wellness for elders. *Holistic Nursing Practice, 7*(1), 38–45.

Walworth, D. (2003). The effect of preferred music genre selection versus preferred song selection on experimentally induced anxiety levels. *Journal of Music Therapy, 40*(1), 2–14.

Waters, M., & Hocker, A. (1991). *Into adolescence: Actions for Wellpower. A curriculum for grades 5–8.* Santa Cruz, CA: Network.

Watt, D., Verma, S., & Flynn, L. (1998). Wellness programs: A review of the evidence. *Canadian Medical Association Journal, 158*(2), 224–230.

White, J., & Nezey, I. O. (1996). Project wellness: A collaborative health promotion program for older adults. *Nursing Connection, 9*, 21–27.

Wilson, R. W., Patterson, M. A., & Alford, D. M. (1989). Services for maintaining independence. *Journal of Gerontological Nursing, 15*(6), 31–37.

Wininger, S. R., & Pargman, D. (2003). Assessment of factors associated with exercise enjoyment. *Journal of Music Therapy, 40*(1), 57–73.

Wolfe, D. E., O'Connell, A. S., & Waldon, E. G. (2002). Music for relaxation: A comparison of musicians and nonmusicians on ratings of selected musical recordings. *Journal of Music Therapy, 39*(1), 40–55.

Chapter 10

Neurologic Music Therapy

Alicia Ann Clair
Varvara Pasiali
Blythe LaGasse

Introduction

The scientific model of Neurologic Music Therapy (NMT) was developed by Dr. Michael Thaut and his colleagues at the Center for Biomedical Research in Music (CBRM) at Colorado State University. Dr. Thaut, a professor of music and professor of neuroscience at Colorado State University, defines Neurologic Music Therapy as "the therapeutic application of music to cognitive, sensory and motor dysfunctions due to neurologic disease of the human nervous system" (Thaut, 1999b, p. 1). It is comprised of a research-based system of standardized clinical techniques for sensorimotor training, speech/language training, and cognitive training in neurologic rehabilitation, neuropediatric therapy, neurogeriatric therapy, and neurodevelopmental therapy. The clinical techniques focus on functional, therapeutic goals in rehabilitation, development, and adaptation. In this chapter, the authors provide an overview of Neurologic Music Therapy and its standardized clinical approaches.

History

Based on the belief that only scientific evidence can establish the acceptance of music therapy among the medical community, researchers at Colorado State University have investigated the effects of music perception and production on nonmusical brain and behavioral functions for the past 15 years (Thaut, 1999b, 2000, 2001). The emergence of Neurologic Music Therapy is based on their continual research findings. Neurologic Music Therapy is, therefore, a research-based system of standardized clinical techniques that provide a framework and structure, based in scientific knowledge, that explain the physiological, neurological, and psychological bases of music therapy (Thaut, 2000). Research demonstrates successful applications in (a) neurologic rehabilitation (with clients who had a cerebralvascular accident [CVA], a traumatic brain injury [TBI], Parkinson's disease, multiple sclerosis, or Huntington's disease); (b) neuropediatric therapy (with clients who have muscular dystrophy, or TBI due to accident, surgery, or disease such as cancer); (c) neurogeriatric therapy (with clients with Alzheimer's disease, other dementias, and Huntington's disease); and (d) neurodevelopmental therapy (with clients who have cerebral palsy, autism, severe visual impairments, or developmental delays). Neurologic music therapists are trained in neuroanatomy, neurophysiology, brain pathology, medical terminology, and rehabilitation of cognitive and motor functions (Thaut, 2001). Training currently takes place at Colorado State University, Fort Collins, which offers both undergraduate and master's degrees and a continuing education training program through the Center for Biomedical Research in Music. Efforts are underway to establish additional training centers nationally and internationally through the Robert F. Unkefer Academy of Neurologic Music Therapy, a professional organization established in 2002 to advance education and understanding of the scientific, evidence-based practice of Neurologic Music Therapy. The academy provides basic and advanced training institutes each year, which offer, respectively, the professional designations of NMT (Neurologic Music Therapist), and Fellow of the Academy. NMT is currently fully integrated into teaching curricula at five other universities in the United States (Western Michigan University, University of Kansas, University of Miami, University of Louisville, Sam Houston State University) and one university in Europe (University of Applied Sciences, Heidelberg, Germany).

Philosophy

The four essential paradigms for Neurologic Music Therapy are: (a) Neuroscience-guided Rehabilitation, (b) Learning and Training Models, (c) Cortical Plasticity Models, and (d) Neurological Facilitation Models (Thaut, 2005). Neuroscience-guided Rehabilitation integrates evidence-based outcomes from brain research and clinical studies. Learning and Training Models illustrate how rhythmic motor learning and training functions in relationship to temporal structure and organization to enhance cognitive, speech, and language functioning. The Cortical Plasticity Models incorporate music as a complex, rhythmically organized, and spectrally diverse sound structure that drives neural patterns, which are influenced by temporal modulations of the sensory input. Neurological Facilitation Models describe how patterned sensory input, consisting of auditory rhythmicity and musical patterns, enhance both motor and cognitive functions. In all four models, the time-based structure of music functions to reorganize synaptic connections (Thaut, 2005).

The Neurologic Music Therapy model aims to provide an understanding of how musical responses can be meaningfully translated into cognitive, affective, and sensorimotor therapeutic responses. To elucidate the translation of the musical therapeutic responses, the CBRM developed the Rational-Scientific Mediating Model (R-SMM) of music therapy, which describes the reciprocal relationship between musical behavior and brain function. This relationship represents a paradigm shift in music therapy from a social science model to a perceptual neuroscience model. Within this model, the therapeutic effect of music is determined by studying the stimulation of the brain as it functions in cognition, speech and language, motor control, and emotion, with concomitant psychological and physiological processes in music perception (Thaut, 2005, p. 116) According to Thaut (2005):

The concept of music as a mediating stimulus leads to the conceptualization of how music engages and then changes behavior. Outcomes of music cognition, music and affective responses, music and sensorimotor process can be documented in scientific data and analyzed for parallel outcomes of nonmusical behaviors. (p. 117)

The R-SMM begins with a close examination of musical and nonmusical theoretical models for clarifying the physiological and psychological foundations of human behavior and perception. Both musical response and nonmusical response exemplars are compared and analyzed to find similarities. Based on the identified similarities between the musical and nonmusical models, mediating models are then formed. The mediating models aim to closely define the affective, cognitive, and sensorimotor influences of music on both healthy and dysfunctional brains. Subsequently, theories and rationales based on the mediating models provide an excellent source for forming future research hypotheses. The mediating models function as a thesaurus for drawing topics for clinical research. Clinical research models focus on identifying carryover effects after treatment and behavioral changes that endure over time. This culminates in the application of the clinical research models in clinical practice (Thaut, 2000).

Thaut (2000, 2005) has developed a five-step model called the Transformational Design Model (TDM) for enabling clinicians to metamorphose the scientific model R-SMM to functional therapeutic applications. The five steps are:

1. Conducting diagnostic, etiological, and functional assessment of the client.
2. Developing appropriate therapeutic goals and measurable objectives.
3. Designing functional, nonmusical therapeutic interventions and stimuli by collaborating across therapy disciplines and creating a person-centered approach; working with members of an interdisciplinary team to achieve the same therapeutic goals.
4. Translating the therapeutic goals, stimuli, and exercises identified by the treatment team into functional, therapeutic music therapy interventions that serve the same goals as the nonmusical therapeutic interventions conducted by other therapists.
5. Transferring therapeutic learning and treatment outcomes to real-world applications.

Regarding the fourth step of the TDM model, there are three principles for translating nonmusical interventions to musical interventions. First, the translation should be based on scientific information developed in the R-SMM. Second, the TDM requires that the therapeutic interventions constitute a musical experience that is aesthetic and artistically pleasing. Finally, "the therapeutic music experience has to be isomorphic in therapeutic structure and function to the general therapy experience" (Thaut, 2000, p. 38). In this effort, the music therapist must implement therapeutic interventions that are pertinent to each client's treatment plan (Thaut, 2000). The Neurologic Music Therapy treatment techniques incorporated into individual treatment plans are research-based and are directed to meet functional therapeutic goals. Treatment techniques are standardized and applied to therapy as therapeutic music interventions (TMI), which are adaptable to the patient's needs. The authors outline the Neurologic Music Therapy techniques in the following section.

Neurologic Therapy Model

The standardized Neurologic Music Therapy interventions are used for three types of training: (a) sensorimotor training, (b) speech and language training, and (c) cognitive training. In this section, the authors list and describe, on an introductory level, the therapeutic mechanisms and goals of each type of training and the applicable neurologic techniques. The definitions and the descriptions for the mechanisms first appeared in the *Training Manual for Neurologic Music Therapy* (Thaut, 1999b) and were revised most recently in 2003. For more information, readers should refer to protocols developed at the Center for Biomedical Research and Music and by members of the Robert F. Unkefer Academy of Neurologic Music Therapy

Sensorimotor Training

Sensorimotor training aims to remediate gait disorders, improve posture, and facilitate upper extremity movement. The therapeutic mechanisms employed include audio-spinal facilitation, sensorimotor integration, rhythmic entrainment, auditory feedback, and patterned information processing, particularly that which deals with sonification (Thaut, 1999b). The standardized techniques used for gait, posture, and arm and trunk training are Rhythmic Auditory Stimulation (RAS), Patterned Sensory Enhancement (PSE), and Therapeutic Instrumental Music Playing (TIMP) (Thaut, 2001).

Rhythmic Auditory Stimulation (RAS)—According to the *NMT Training Manual* (Thaut, 1999b), RAS is a technique that facilitates movements that are intrinsically rhythmical in a repetitive pattern, such as gait. This technique uses music as an external time cue to regulate the body's movement in time. With RAS, the therapist assesses the gait parameters of a client and matches the ambulation speed with a rhythmic cue using a metronome or another device. The rhythmic cue is embedded into background music to facilitate engagement. The client then performs gait-training exercises while listening to the rhythmic auditory stimulation. The external rhythmic cue organizes motor responses and, as a result, improves functional motor outcomes (Thaut, 1999b). While RAS is used almost exclusively in stroke rehabilitation, potential applications include those with children who have developmental disabilities, adults who are physically frail, persons with late stage dementia, and others.

Patterned Sensory Enhancement (PSE)—PSE is defined as "a technique using rhythmic, melodic, harmonic and dynamic-acoustical elements of music to provide temporal, spatial and force patterns to structure and cue functional movements" (Thaut, 1999b). PSE can be used to structure both rhythmical and discrete movements in the arms, hands, upper trunk, or entire body. Applications of PSE incorporate individual musical patterns in which rhythm structures the timing, duration guides the range of motion, pitch indicates direction in space, and dynamics and harmony direct the amount of force of separate movements. These musical patterns are incorporated into a series to guide movements into sequences that form functional movement patterns, such as the extension of an arm to reach and the closure of the hand to grasp. PSE is broader in application than RAS because it (a) facilitates movements that are not rhythmical by nature (e.g., hand and arm movements required for eating, dressing, and other ADLs, as well as whole body movements required to shift from a seated to a standing position); and (b) provides a broad range of cues, not just temporal cues (Thaut, 1999b).

Therapeutic Instrumental Music Playing (TIMP)—TIMP is defined as the use of musical instrument playing to facilitate engagement in physical exercise and to simulate functional movement patterns in motor therapy. In TIMP, musical instruments are selected for their therapeutic potential and are positioned for playing to facilitate increased range of motion, endurance, strength, functional hand movements and finger dexterity, and motor coordination. Musical accompaniments are used to provide structure for the movements.

Speech and Language Training

The neurologic music therapist may implement several techniques to remediate speech and language deficits or to maintain language in patients with debilitating conditions such as dementia or Parkinson's disease. The therapeutic mechanisms involved in the treatment include differential hemispheric processing, patterned information processing, perceptual sensory priming, and rhythmic entrainment (Thaut, 1999b). The standardized techniques include Melodic Intonation Therapy (MIT), Musical Speech Stimulation (MUSTIM), Rhythmic Speech Cueing (RSC), Vocal Intonation Therapy (VIT), Therapeutic Singing (TS), Oral Motor and Respiratory Exercises (OMREX), Developmental Speech and Language Training Through Music (DSLM), and Symbolic Communication Training Through Music (SYCOM) (Thaut, 2001).

Melodic Intonation Therapy (MIT)—This technique is used for persons with expressive aphasia, with some evidence of success with persons who have apraxia. It is based on a protocol developed by Sparks and Holland (1976) that incorporates an individual's unimpaired ability to sing to facilitate spontaneous and voluntary speech. This technique uses functional phrases that are initially sung in prosody and intonation similar to spoken words; then the phrases are incorporated into "speech singing," followed by the spoken phrase produced with normal speech characteristics.

Musical Speech Stimulation (MUSTIM)—The purpose of this technique is to produce nonpropositional speech in persons who have aphasia. The technique incorporates initiation or completion of overlearned songs, chants, rhymes, and musical phrases to elicit spoken words or functional phrases (Basso, Capatini, & Vignolo, 1979). For example, when presented with overlearned song lyrics, an individual is likely to fill in the blank, such as "You are my_____" (Thaut, 1999b).

Rhythmic Speech Cuing (RSC)—This technique is beneficial for clients who have apraxia, dysarthria, and fluency disorders. It employs rhythmic cues that control the rate of speech as well as speech initiation. To illustrate, hand tapping or drum playing is initiated at a tempo compatible with appropriate speech prosody before the speech is attempted. Once the rhythmic structure is in place, the individual is asked to initiate speech. The ongoing tapping or drumming during the subsequent speech provides the temporal structure to control the speech rate (Thaut, 1999b). This technique is also effective with clients with low intellectual ability (Thaut, 2001).

Vocal Intonation Therapy (VIT)—The goal of VIT is to train elements of vocal control, including inflection, pitch, breath control, timbre, and loudness. VIT differs from MIT in that it is used to enhance functional speech affected by voice disorders, not to initially develop the speech. In VIT clients learn exercises in which sung phrases simulate the prosody, inflection, and pace of typical speech. The sung phrases are faded to spoken phrases. This technique is often used with clients who speak with a monotone voice as a result of a traumatic brain injury and with those who have voice disorders (Thaut, 1999b, 2001).

Therapeutic Singing (TS)—This technique, which facilitates rehabilitation for persons with a range of neurological and/or developmental speech and language dysfunctions, uses singing to initiate and develop speech, improve articulation, and increase respiratory function. For example, singing is used during early stages of rehabilitation following trauma to strengthen muscles, to initiate and trigger sound production, and to increase breath control and posture (Thaut, 1999b, 2001). This technique is applicable with various clinical populations. One example is the use of TS with persons who have Parkinson's disease to strengthen vocal production.

Oral Motor and Respiratory Exercises (OMREX)—To achieve better sound vocalization, improved articulation, increased respiratory strength, and better speech mechanism function, OMREX employs musical wind instrument playing and oral exercise performances (Thaut, 1999b). For instance, oral motor exercises inherent in wind instrument playing are used to strengthen the mouth musculature (Thaut, 2001). The breath support required when playing a wind instrument functions to increase respiratory capacity.

Developmental Speech and Language Training Through Music (DSLM)—DSLM functions to develop initial speech and language through singing, chanting, playing musical instruments, and combinations of music, speech, and movement (Thaut, 1999b). This technique is successful with children who have little to no functional language, such as children with autism and children with other developmental disabilities.

Symbolic Communication Training Through Music (SYCOM)—This technique employs structured musical performances and/or improvisational musical performances. Performances involve instrumental music making, vocal music making, or both. The goal is to achieve behaviors inherent in communication (Thaut, 1999b). The music playing experiences provide opportunities to learn communication skills that are similar to the skills required in verbal and nonverbal social interactions, such as listening, question/answer responses, statements, and waiting for input, among others.

Cognitive Training

Cognitive training is essential for clients who have developmental disabilities, autism, attention deficit disorder, attention hyperactivity disorder, traumatic brain injury, or other socioemotional deficits. Cognitive training is divided into four subcategories: (a) auditory attention and perception training, (b) memory training, (c) executive function training, and (d) psychosocial behavior training (Thaut, 2001).

Subcategory 1. Auditory Attention and Perception Training

The standardized therapeutic techniques include Music Sensory Orientation Training (MSOT), Musical Neglect Training (MNT), Auditory Perception Training (APT), and Musical Attention Control Training (MACT) (Thaut, 2001). The therapeutic mechanisms involved with these training techniques include patterned information processing, perceptual sensory priming, attention to rhythm, and auditory information processing (Thaut, 1999b).

Musical Sensory Orientation Training (MSOT)—This technique is used with individuals who have severe to profound developmental disabilities or with patients who are comatose (Thaut,

2001). The application of the technique begins with sensory stimulation, where live or recorded music is used to evoke arousal responses. It moves to arousal orientation, where the person orients to person, place, and time, and eventually progresses to vigilance and attention maintenance, where the focus is initially on the quantity, not on the quality of ongoing attention that is incorporated into active music engagement in music (Thaut, 1999b).

Musical Neglect Training (MNT)—MNT is used with clients with one-side sensory weakness that results from trauma and who have sensory processing deficits with stimuli presented to the affected side (Thaut, 2001). MNT incorporates rhythmically structured instrumental music playing that requires the individual to focus attention in the neglected or unattended visual field. In this approach, rhythm percussion instruments are positioned to require the individual to use the neglected visual field to play them. An alternative to this approach is one that incorporates an auditory presentation of music to stimulate hemispheric brain processing concomitantly with participation in exercises designed to remediate visual neglect or inattention (Thaut, 1999b).

Auditory Perception Training (APT)—APT requires individuals to discriminate among sounds and to identify sound components that include time, tempo, duration, pitch, timbre, rhythmic patterns, and speech sounds (Thaut, 1999b). For example, rhythm and pitched instruments are used to provide the stimulus for discrimination. Here clients indicate through playing or listening which instruments are faster, sound higher/lower, have the longest sound, are the loudest, and are played in the same rhythmic pattern as a spoken phrase, and so on. Furthermore, APT requires individuals to integrate sensory stimuli, which include those that are auditory, tactile, visual, and kinesthetic, such as reading symbols or notes that direct music instrumental playing, moving or dancing with music, or feeling tactile sensations of sound while beating a drum.

Musical Attention Control Training (MACT)—MACT includes active or receptive participation in which music that is either composed or improvised cues one of four different types of attention: (a) selective, (b) sustained, (c) divided, and (d) alternating (Thaut, 1999b). The neurologic music therapist implements applications designed to improve different types of attention skills according to individual client needs. Selective attention applications aim to teach a client how to focus attention on a single sensory source and ignore other sensory elements in the environment. Sustained attention is designed to maintain focus of attention, and to increase the duration of attention focus for progressively longer periods. Divided attention applications teach clients to focus on two different sensory sources at the same time, whereas alternating attention applications teach a client to shift attention from one source of stimulation to another (Thaut, 2001).

Subcategory 2. Memory Training

Memory training includes therapeutic mechanisms of patterned information processing using Gestalt principles, affect modification, and applications of the associative network theory of mood and memory (CBRM, 1999). The standardized therapeutic techniques include Musical Mnemonics Training (MMT) and Associative Mood and Memory Training (AMMT) (Thaut, 2001).

Musical Mnemonics Training (MMT)—This technique is used for memory training where music is used to stimulate encoding and decoding/recall functions (Thaut, 1999b). There are three different types of mnemonic exercises: (a) echoing mnemonics, (b) procedural mnemonics, and (c) declarative mnemonics. Echoing mnemonics applications emphasize immediate recall of sensory information. Procedural mnemonic applications deal with remembering rules and previously learned skills. On the other hand, declarative mnemonics applications teach semantic and episodic memory skills, pertaining to decoding symbolic information (Thaut, 2001). In all three types of mnemonics, songs, rhymes, or chants are used to provide the structure in which nonmusical information is presented sequentially and where it can be organized into "chunks" to enhance the learning experience.

Associative Mood and Memory Training (AMMT)—AMMT is based on the facilitation of moods or emotional states that can have three purposes: (a) to establish a mood that is likely to facilitate recall; (b) to evoke a mood that is associated with memory and, therefore, provides direct access to the memory; and (c) to induce a positive mood, or emotional state, that is conducive to learning and recall (Thaut, 1999b). With the first two purposes, AMMT is predicated on the past experiences of a client and the mood state in which learning took place. With AMMT, the recall of previously learned material has greater potential for recall when the mood in which it was originally learned is reinstated (Thaut, 2001). In addition, new learning and recall is more likely to occur when a positive mood is established prior to the learning attempt.

Subcategory 3. Executive Function Training

Executive function training is based on therapeutic mechanisms that include patterned information processing that uses Gestalt principles and social learning (Thaut, 1999b). The standardized therapeutic technique is Musical Executive Function Training (MEFT) (Thaut, 2001).

Musical Executive Function Training (MEFT)—MEFT uses musical improvisations and compositions in either group or individual sessions to provide practice with executive function skills, including organization, problem solving, decision making, reasoning, and comprehension Music performances provide the context for using the skills within a sensory structure that organizes temporal responses, accommodates creative expression, allows appropriate emotional expression, and supports social interactions (Thaut, 1999b).

Subcategory 4. Psychosocial Behavior Training

Psychosocial behavior training relies on the therapeutic mechanisms of affect modification, classical conditioning, operant conditioning, and social learning, along with applications of associative network theory of mood and memory (Thaut, 1999b). The standardized therapeutic technique is Music Psychotherapy and Counseling (MPC) (Thaut, 2001).

Music Psychotherapy and Counseling (MPC)—MPC includes a wide range of music uses to (a) induce and change moods, (b) provide cognitive reorientation, (c) train affective behavior responses, (d) train social skills, and (e) provide musical incentive training for behavior modification. Music applications include, among others, guided listening and active music making with composed and improvised music. Music involvement leads to appropriate emotional expressions; social interactions; and orientation to person, time, and place; along with opportunities to develop impulse control and mood management that facilitate improved psychosocial functions (Thaut, 1999b).

Neurologic Music Therapy Research

There are many theories regarding time perception and discrimination by humans (Tecchio, Salustri, Thaut, Pasqualetti, & Rossini, 2000). Magnetoencephalographic (MEG) measurements have indicated that humans have the ability to process information regarding rhythmic variations of auditory stimuli, even when these are not consciously identifiable. These measurements imply the existence of connections between auditory and motor cortexes in the human brain (Tecchio et al., 2000), and the effect of rhythm on physical movement entrainment and coordination has long been evident. Music cannot exist without rhythmic organization, and rhythmic music enables humans to synchronize their movements by dancing, clapping, or toe tapping. Advances in technology have allowed researchers to investigate the role of rhythm as an internalized timekeeper for motoric movements (Thaut, 1999b).

Several studies indicated that rhythmic auditory stimulation (RAS) affects stride parameters and EMG patterns of healthy adults. In one study, RAS improved stride rhythmicity and affected muscle activity by increasing efficiency of motoric patterns (Thaut, McIntosh, Prassas, & Rice, 1992). Other studies indicated that rhythmic cuing influenced the EMG patterns of upper extremity muscles during a motor activity (Thaut, Schleiffers, & Davis, 1991) and improved synchronization of finger tapping (Thaut, Rathbun, & Miller, 1997; Thaut, Tian, & Azimi-Sadjadi, 1998). In addition, rhythmic cueing was used with cellists who daily practiced a specific playing technique that involved rapid left-hand successions. Changes in EMG patterns indicated that rhythmic cueing facilitated the performance of the motor movements associated with playing techniques that led to an enhanced performance (Thiem, Green, Prassas, & Thaut, 1994). Other scientific studies have investigated the role of RAS in therapeutic interventions.

Research in laboratory settings has shown that Rhythmic Auditory stimulation (RAS) training increases movement coordination of clients suffering from neurological motor problems as a result of a cerebralvascular accident (CVA, stroke), Parkinson's disease, TBI, Huntington's disease, Alzheimer's disease, spinal cord injury, and cerebral palsy. Studies indicated that after 3 to 5 weeks of RAS gait training, the patient's gait performance improved in cadence, velocity, stride length, and gait symmetry; the variability of electromyography (EMG) activation patterns was reduced (Hurt, Rice, McIntosh, & Thaut, 1998). After participating in a 3-week therapy program consisting of walking using RAS stimulation, patients with Parkinson's disease displayed electromyographic (EMG) gait-cycle profiles that approximated normal EMG gait patterns (Miller, Thaut, McIntosh, & Rice, 1996). Moreover, as a result of gait entrainment using RAS training, patients with Parkinson's disease taking medication showed a 36% increase in gait velocity. Patients who had not taken any medication showed a 25% velocity increase. Both groups achieved a 10% increase in cadence (McIntosh, Brown, Rice, & Thaut, 1997). Other studies have demonstrated increase in gait performance during functional in-home tasks with rhythmic auditory stimulation (Nieuwboer et al., 2007; Rochester et al., 2005). One study showed that, unlike those with Parkinson's disease, persons with Huntington's disease did not respond well to musical cues for motor timing and movement synchronization, yet they increased their gait velocity following metronome cuing. This was likely due to decreased cognitive capacities characteristic of the Huntington's disease process (Thaut, Miltner, Lang, Hurt, & Hoemberg, 1999). In another study, an experimental and control group of patients with hemiparetic stroke underwent a 6-week, twice-daily gait-training program. The control group participated in a traditional physical therapy gait program, whereas the experimental group was trained using the same traditional program with the addition of RAS. As an external timekeeper, RAS was used to entrain and gradually synchronize step patterns. Pre- and posttests indicated that the patients of the RAS group, compared with the control group, had a statistically significant increase in velocity (164% vs. 107%), stride length (88% vs. 34%), and reduction in EMG amplitude variability of the gastrocnemius muscle (69% vs. 33%). Both groups had improved stride symmetry, 32% for the RAS group and 16% for the control group; the difference between the two groups was not significant (Thaut, McIntosh, & Rice, 1997). When comparing two types of gait training with patients with hemiparetic stroke over a period of 3 weeks, Thaut et al. (2007) found that those patients assigned in the RAS group improved significantly. Improvement in gait parameters was significantly higher for the patients in RAS group in comparison to the patients assigned in the other treatment condition.

A preliminary clinical study of 15 persons in late-stage Alzheimer's disease showed that individuals have higher velocities and longer stride length with RAS than without (Clair & O'Konski, 2001). In addition, persons in late-stage Alzheimer's disease had significantly greater engagement in exercises that included RAS than with the same exercises without RAS (Mathews, Clair, & Kosloski, 2001). Ogata (2006) studied the clinical use of RAS with frail elderly and found RAS treatment increased walking distance, velocity, and stride length. Additional studies indicated that RAS significantly reduced knee tremor in a group of five patients with gait hemiparesis as a result of TBI (Kenyon & Thaut, 2000), and improved gait parameters of children with cerebral palsy (Kwak, 2000) and patients with incomplete spinal cord injury (de l'Etoile, 2008). Conclusively, RAS can be effective as a therapeutic enhancement to traditional treatment.

Research also substantiates the benefits of Neurologic Music Therapy techniques in speech and language rehabilitation. In a pilot study, Pilon, McIntosh, and Thaut (1998) compared using auditory and visual speech timing cues for reducing speech rate and increasing speech intelligibility in three males with dysarthric impairments resulting from TBI. The results indicated that the two participants who had the most severe speech impairments were able to synchronize their speech with the rhythmic cues, decrease speech rate, and, as a result, improve speech intelligibility. In another study examining the effects of rhythmic speech cueing on speech intelligibility in 20 patients with Parkinson's disease, speech cueing generated the most substantial results in patients with severe speech impairments. The speech of patients with moderate impairment was slightly improved. There was no benefit for patients with mild impairments (Thaut, McIntosh, McIntosh, & Hoemberg, 2001). Clinical research with four patients diagnosed with Parkinson's disease showed significant increases in speech intelligibility and vocal intensity following a series of 12 to 14 sessions of engagement in a therapeutic singing protocol. Subjects in this study also indicated elevated mood, likely as a result of their speech intelligibility and vocal intensity improvements (Haneishi, 2002). Other researchers studied using Neurologic Music Therapy techniques for speech and language with children who have developmental disorders. For example, Lim (2007) examined the effect of Developmental Speech and Language (DSLM) therapeutic applications with children who have autism spectrum diagnoses. DSLM improved speech production, particularly with children who were lower functioning.

There is ample scientific evidence regarding Neurologic Music Therapy and cognitive training. Music used to induce mood prior to learning and recall significantly enhanced the ability to recall information (Thaut & de l'Etoile, 1993). Listening to preferred relaxing music decreased state anxiety measures and increased relaxation responses of college students (Davis & Thaut, 1989; Thaut & Davis, 1993). Moreover, participation in music therapy interventions produced positive self-rated changes in relaxation, affect, and thought processes in 50 male psychiatric-prisoner patients (Thaut, 1989). Research has also verified the effectiveness of music as a mnemonic device (Claussen & Thaut, 1997; Gfeller, 1983; Wallace, 1994). A study that examined retention of multiplication tables for 21 children with learning disabilities indicated that familiar music rehearsal resulted in higher average recall accuracy than verbal rehearsal (Claussen & Thaut, 1997). Furthermore, music as a mnemonic device has been shown to increase word order memory in persons with memory deficits due to multiple sclerosis (McIntosh, Peterson, & Thaut, 2006; Thaut, Peterson, & McIntosh, 2005; Thaut, Peterson, Sena, & McIntosh, 2008). Studebaker (2007) examined the use of a music therapy protocol for attention retraining with four patients who had stroke. The patients had improved neuropsychosocial evaluation scores. They also self-reported improved cognitive functioning. The following section includes a short description of Neurologic Music Therapy applications.

Music Therapy Applications

All applications of Neurologic Music Therapy are taught at the Center for Biomedical Research in Music and through the Robert F. Unkefer Academy of Neurologic Music Therapists. The selected applications described here provide some basic information, but are not a substitute for the detailed training necessary for clinical practice applications.

Sensorimotor Training Applications

RAS is the most researched of the Neurologic Music Therapy applications. The purpose of RAS is to use rhythm to improve gait velocity and symmetry, to modify stride length, and to improve step cadence. It occurs in a three-step process: (a) pre-gait exercise, (b) gait training, and (c) advanced gait training. RAS can also be applied to rhythmically organized movements other than gait, including repetitive training of upper limb motions, such as elbow flexions and extensions, or arm swings (Thaut, 1999b).

Pre-gait exercises include forward and backward weight transfers, and side to side weight transfers while standing between parallel bars. In addition, they consist of seated exercises including knee extensions, marching, and rising from a seated to a standing position (Thaut 1999b). The initial gait training is performed in five steps: (a) assessment, (b) resonant frequency entrainment, (c) frequency modulation, (d) fading, and (e) reassessment. Advanced gait training involves ambulation on a variety of surfaces, up and down stairs, and around obstacles with shifts in direction, as well as opportunities to stop and go (Thaut, 1999b).

The clinical applications for persons with Parkinson's disease or traumatic brain injury due to cerebral vascular accident focus on increased walking speed with improved stability. The approach involves a careful study of the gait characteristics and an assessment of the cadence (the number of steps per minute), the velocity (the number of meters per minute), and the stride length (velocity divided by cadence times two). The clinical applications for persons in late-stage dementia and other diseases, such as Huntington's disease, are designed to meet the goal for maintenance of ambulation with good stability. Careful assessment of gait characteristics remains the basis of the treatment, and no efforts are made to speed the gait. The goal is to maintain ambulation for as long as possible into the debilitating disease process. It is likely that persons who experience Rhythmic Auditory Stimulation (RAS) can maintain their ambulation further into the disease process than those persons who do not have the treatment; however, the research to support this hypothesis is currently untested.

Therapeutic Instrumental Music Playing (TIMP) involves playing musical instruments in ways that stimulate movements that are functional. Individual programs are targeted on relearning functional movement skills; overcoming unhealthy compensation strategies; and increasing strength, endurance, and range of motion (Thaut, 1999b). This could involve reaching from side to side to play a drum, or reaching across the midline to strike a tambourine. It may also involve using a musical instrument as a target to delimit the range of motion in an exercise, that is, extending the knee while seated until the toe of the shoe makes contact with a jingle stick, or moving fingers in pincher grasp to play finger cymbals. Whatever the movement, a musical instrument is used as a sound stimulus to achieve goals of increased range of motion, endurance, functional hand movements, finger dexterity, and limb coordination. Therefore, instruments may be used in traditional ways for positioning and playing, or may be altered in either positioning or playing to facilitate a desired response (Thaut, 1999b).

Patterned Sensory Enhancement (PSE) uses music to reflect the movement structure so that the music "fits" the movement pattern that is practiced with it (Thaut, 1999b). The therapist begins by conceptualizing the movement pattern, then illustrates the pattern through the music, and includes the desired movement pattern into a music therapy exercise. PSE can be used to facilitate simple movements, such as an arm flexion and extension exercise, or more complicated movement patterns, such as reaching for, grasping, and lifting an object (Thaut, 2005).

Speech and Language Training Applications

The Neurologic Music Therapy clinical applications of Melodic Intonation Therapy (MIT) are based on the model developed by Sparks and Holland (1976). The NMT applications differ, however, in the length of the phrases trained. The NMT approach lengthens the phrases to allow better opportunities for entrainment. Success in the speech training using MIT is facilitated not only by the melodic contour, but also by the rhythm of the phrases.

Haneishi (2002) developed and tested a protocol to enhance speech intelligibility and other vocal characteristics of persons with Parkinson's disease using Therapeutic Singing (TS). Her protocol consisted of (a) 3 minutes of opening conversation; (b) 5 minutes of warm-up including facial massage, facial muscle exercises, and inhalation/exhalation exercises; (c) 20 minutes of vocal exercises including those to warm-up the laryngeal musculature, promote deep breathing, increase resonance, increase breath support, increase resonance, and improve articulation; (d) 15 minutes of singing using preferred songs; (e) 5 minutes of vowel phonation; (f) 9 minutes of speech exercise review; and (g) closing conversation. The protocol yielded significant improvements in speech intelligibility and vocal intensity, along with increased measures of positive mood.

Controlling the rate of speech with Rhythmic Speech Cueing (RSC) has been effective with persons who have dysarthria (Pilon et al., 1998). This technique emphasizes controlling the rate of speech production, which can improve intelligibility. In RSC, the rate of the pacing cue has been shown to impact the success of the technique (Thaut et al., 2001). The rhythmic cues either can be evenly distributed (metric) or can follow the natural stress of the phrase (patterned). Concurrently playing an instrument, such as a drum, while speaking can be used to further reinforce the pattern of the phrase.

Developmental Speech and Language Training Through Music (DSLM) can be utilized to engage children in therapeutic experiences focused on improving verbal communication and use of language. Applications are extremely experiential with developmentally appropriate language learning integrated into the experience. Multimodal stimulation can be used to reinforce learning with a combination of music, movement, and visual aids. The focus in DSLM is not simply imitation or repetition of phrases, rather learning of speech and language through the use of and exposure to developmentally appropriate language. This process may also involve focused practice of specific articulations that are then transferred into appropriate words through a motivating and age-appropriate experience.

Cognitive Training Applications

There are several applications that facilitate cognitive training. An example of an echoing mnemonics application is for the therapist to play two notes on the keyboard and ask the client if they sounded the same or different. A procedural mnemonics exercise would be to play a simple chord procession on the keyboard, wait, and then play again; the client should identify if the progression was the same or if it changed. Declarative mnemonics applications involve analyzing and remembering the content of songs (Thaut, 2001).

An example of a selective attention application is for the therapist to ask a client to focus his or her attention on what the therapist plays on the piano. Then the therapist asks the client to play a drum only when the therapist plays on the high register of the piano. An application to train sustained attention is exemplified when the therapist asks the client to play a drum to accompany the improvisational music that the therapist plays on the keyboard. When the client listens to a musical pattern that was identified and learned before the application began, the client is directed to stop playing the drum and to resume only when the therapist finishes playing the musical pattern and continues with improvisation.

Applications for musical executive function training may include playing musical compositional games using a variety of instruments. The therapist may choose to use a software program, play examples of rhythmic patterns or instrumental sounds for the client, ask the client to choose what she or he likes, and gradually develop a music composition.

Neurologic Music Therapy for Children

Neurologic music therapy techniques can be utilized to address functional goals in children with neurological disabilities, developmental disabilities, or autism. According to Thaut (1999a), major areas of focus with children who have disabilities include education, rehabilitation, and development. Education includes academic skills, such as learning numbers and colors. Rehabilitative goals focus on restoration of skills that have been lost due to injury.

Developmental goals enhance the course of normal development by providing social, emotional, and sensorimotor experiences (Thaut, 1999a).

In order to properly utilize NMT techniques with children, it is essential to understand brain development, as neurological development in children is different from neurological rehabilitation in adults. Furthermore, children who are developing skills for the first time may require some different strategies from children who are relearning a previously mastered skill. Therefore, a protocol developed for rehabilitation may not transfer to the developmental model. Careful consideration of neurological development, in addition to an understanding of the natural development of sensorimotor, communication, and social skills, is essential to providing quality services.

Children have different abilities in motor entrainment than adults. Research has demonstrated that children under five years of age do not match an external stimulus (Sloboda, 1985). Rhythmic entrainment to an auditory stimulus may not be realistic when treating children with developmental disabilities (Hurt-Thaut & Johnson, 2003). However, the ability to entrain intrinsic motor movement to an external stimulus has been demonstrated in preterm infants who entrain to a tactile rhythmic stimulus for nonnutritive suck and rhythmic breathing (Barlow & Estep, 2006; Ingersoll & Thoman, 1994). These studies show that children have the ability to entrain to an external stimulus; however, there is a need for more research on auditory entrainment for both intrinsic and volitional tasks in children.

Several research studies have demonstrated the effectiveness of NMT techniques with children. Rhythmic Auditory Stimulation (RAS) has been successful in improving gait velocity, stride length, and stability in children with cerebral palsy (Hurt et al., 1997; Kwak, 2000). Melodic intonation therapy (MIT) has been effective in the treatment of children with developmental apraxia of speech (Helfrich-Miller, 1984; Krauss & Galloway, 1982). Children with learning disabilities have shown increased learning with musical mnemonics training (Claussen & Thaut, 1997). Pasiali (2008) demonstrated the benefit of cognitive training with NMT techniques for building resiliency skills of children in home-based settings. These selected research studies are just a few examples of how NMT techniques can be effective in the treatment of children.

The NMT model provides the music therapist with the scientific foundation, the framework to create therapeutic music exercises that are transferable to nonmusical outcomes, and an extensive list of techniques that can be used with many different populations. While the use of several NMT techniques has been effective in the treatment of children, careful consideration of the child's developmental level is essential for quality treatment.

Conclusion

The scientific model for Neurologic Music Therapy is well established. The most researched area is Rhythmic Auditory Stimulation (RAS), where the laboratory research is extensive, and research of clinical applications is currently underway in many populations. Though RAS is essential to rehabilitation and the maintenance of functional behaviors in sensorimotor training, Therapeutic Instrumental Music Performance (TIMP) and Patterned Sensory Enhancement (PSE) are also integral to gait and posture training and arm and trunk training in rehabilitation and habilitation.

A second area of Neurologic Music Therapy, speech and language training, is under development with the majority of the published outcomes in Auditory Speech Cueing and Therapeutic Singing. Though applications of Melodic Intonation Therapy are traditionally applied to individuals who have suffered damage to Brocca's area of the brain, applications in the future may be extended to other populations, including children with developmental apraxia of speech. Therapeutic Singing is viable with a wide range of persons with vocal disorders, and further research is planned to expand its application with persons who have Parkinson's disease.

Cognitive training, the third area of Neurologic Music Therapy, is extensive with applications in wide ranges of populations. Music therapists have practiced in many of these populations in the past without benefit of laboratory and clinical research that validates their applications. In this area, and all areas of music therapy practice, it is necessary to gain an understanding of how music responses are meaningfully translated into therapeutic responses.

The research to fully understand music therapy interventions is a monumental task. It can be based in Thaut's conceptualization of a comprehensive model that includes affective, cognitive, and sensorimotor behaviors through four progressively more complex levels that include: (a) musical responses to basic music perception and music performance; (b) comparisons of musical and nonmusical behaviors in the same, or parallel, contexts; (c) studies of the effects of musical responses on nonmusical behaviors; and (d) clinical models that draw from the research of the influence of music on nonmusical behaviors and systematically test the outcomes of applications in music therapy treatment (Thaut, 2000, p. 48).

The research and clinical practice models designed and tested in Neurologic Music Therapy have established music therapy in rehabilitation. Research outcomes have validated the therapeutic applications of music in a range of populations. Future research will establish Neurologic Music Therapy throughout the therapeutic field.

References

Barlow, S., & Estep, M. (2006). Central pattern generation and the motor infrastructure for suck, respiration, and speech. *Journal of Communication Disorders, 39*(5), 366–380.

Basso, A., Capatini, E., & Vignolo, L. A. (1979). Influence of rehabilitation on language skills in aphasic patients. *Archives of Neurology, 36,* 190–196.

Center for Biomedical Research in Music (CBRM). (1999). *Training manual for Neurologic Music Therapy.* Fort Collins, CO: Colorado State University.

Clair, A. A., & O'Konski, M. (2001). Preliminary study of Rhythmic Auditory Stimulation (RAS) in persons who are in late dementia. In A. Clair, M. Thaut, & C. Thaut (Co-Chairs), *Neurologic Music Therapy: Neuroscientific model and evidence-based clinical practice.* Symposium conducted at the annual meeting of the American Music Therapy Association, Pasadena, CA.

Claussen, D. W., & Thaut, M. H. (1997). Music as a mnemonic device for children with learning disabilities. *Canadian Journal of Music Therapy, 5,* 55–66.

Davis, W. B., & Thaut, M. H. (1989). The influence of preferred relaxing music on measures of state anxiety, relaxation, and physiological responses. *Journal of Music Therapy, 26,* 168–187.

de l'Etoile, S. K. (2008). The effect of rhythmic auditory stimulation on the gait parameters of patients with incomplete spinal cord injury: An exploratory pilot study. *International Journal of Rehabilitation*

Research, 31(2), 155. Retrieved May 24, 2008, from Health Module database. (Document ID: 1480898941).

Gfeller, K. E. (1983). Musical mnemonics as an aid to retention with normal and learning disabled students. *Journal of Music Therapy, 20*, 179–189.

Haneishi, E. (2002). Effects of a music therapy voice protocol on speech intelligibility, vocal acoustic measures, and mood of individuals with Parkinson's disease. *Journal of Music Therapy, 38*, 273–290.

Helfrich-Miller, K. R. (1984). Melodic intonation therapy with developmentally apraxic children. *Seminars in Speech and Language, 5*, 119–126.

Hurt, C. P., Rice, R. R., McIntosh, G. C., & Thaut, M. H. (1998). Rhythmic auditory stimulation in gait training for patients with traumatic brain injury. *Journal of Music Therapy, 35*, 228–241.

Hurt-Thaut, C., & Johnson, S. (2003). Neurologic music therapy with children: Scientific foundations and clinical application. In S. Robb (Ed.), *Music therapy in pediatric heathcare: Research and evidence-based practice* (pp. 81–100). Silver Spring, MD: American Music Therapy Association.

Ingersoll, E. W., & Thoman, E. B. (1994). The breathing bear: Effects on respiration in premature infants. *Physiology & Behavior, 56*(5), 855–859.

Kenyon, G. P., & Thaut, M. H. (2000). A measure of kinematic limb instability modulation by rhythmic auditory stimulation. *Journal of Biomechanics, 33*, 1319–1323.

Krauss, T., & Galloway, H. (1982). Melodic Intonation Therapy with language delayed apraxic children. *Journal of Music Therapy, 19*(2), 102–113.

Kwak, E. E. (2000). *Effect of rhythmic auditory stimulation on gait performance in children with spastic cerebral palsy.* Unpublished master's thesis, University of Kansas, Lawrence.

Lim, H. A. (2007). *The effect of "Developmental Speech-Language Training Through Music" on speech production in children with autism spectrum disorders.* (Doctoral dissertation, University of Miami, 2007). Retrieved May 24, 2008, from Dissertations & Theses: A&I database. (Publication No. AAT 3295184)

Mathews, R. M., Clair, A. A., & Kosloski, K. (2001). Keeping the beat: Use of rhythmic music during exercise activities for the elderly with dementia. *American Journal of Alzheimer's Disease and Other Dementias, 16*, 377–380.

McIntosh, G. C, Brown, S. H., Rice, R. R., & Thaut, M. H. (1997). Rhythmic auditory-motor facilitation of gait patterns in patients with Parkinson's disease. *Journal of Neurology, Neurosurgery and Psychiatry, 62*, 22–26.

McIntosh, G. C., Peterson, D. A., & Thaut, M. H. (2006). Verbal learning with a musical template increases neuronal synchronization and improves verbal memory in patients with multiple sclerosis. *Neurorehabilitation & Neural Repair, 20*, 129.

Miller, R. A., Thaut, M. H., McIntosh, G. C., & Rice, R. R. (1996). Components of EMG symmetry and variability in Parkinsonian and healthy elderly gait. *Electroencephalography and Clinical Neurophysiology, 101*, 1–7.

Nieuwboer, A., Kwakkel, G., Rochester, L., Jones, D., van Wegen, E., Willems, A., et al. (2007). Cueing training in the home improves gait-related mobility in Parkinson's disease: The RESCUE trial. *Journal of Neurology, Neurosurgery & Psychiatry, 78*, 134–140.

Ogata, M. (2006). *The effect of rhythmic auditory stimulation on walking distance in the frail elderly.* Unpublished master's thesis. University of Kansas, Lawrence.

Pasiali, V. (2008). *Music therapy and resiliency: A pilot project.* Unpublished manuscript, Michigan State University, East Lansing.

Pilon, M. A., McIntosh, K. W., & Thaut, M. H. (1998). Auditory versus visual speech timing cues as external rate control to enhance verbal intelligibility in mixed spastic-ataxic dysarthric speakers: A pilot study. *Brain Injury, 12,* 793–803.

Rochester, L., Hetherington, V., Jones, D., Nieuwboer, A., Willems, A. M., Kwakkel, G., & Van Wegen, E. (2005). The effect of external rhythmic cues (auditory and visual) on walking during a functional task in homes of people with Parkinson's disease. *Archives of Physical Medicine & Rehabilitation, 86*(5), 999–1006.

Sloboda, J. A. (1985). *The musical mind: The cognitive psychology of music.* Oxford, England: Clarendon Press.

Sparks, R. W., & Holland, A. L. (1976). Method: Melodic intonation therapy for aphasia. *Journal of Speech and Hearing Disorders, 41,* 287–297.

Studebaker, S. E. (2007). *The effect of a music therapy protocol on the attentional abilities of stroke patients.* Unpublished master's thesis. University of Kansas, Lawrence.

Tecchio, F., Salustri, C., Thaut, M. H., Pasqualetti, P., & Rossini, P. M. (2000). Conscious and preconscious adaptation to rhythmic auditory stimuli: A magnetoencephalographic study of human brain responses. *Experimental Brain Research, 135,* 222–230.

Thaut, M. H. (1989). The influence of music therapy interventions on self-rated changes in relaxation, affect, and thought in psychiatric prisoner-patients. *Journal of Music Therapy, 26,* 155–166.

Thaut, M. H. (1999a). Music for children with physical disabilities. In W. B. Davis, K. E. Gfeller, & M. H. Thaut (Eds.), *An introduction to music therapy: Theory and practice* (2nd ed.; pp. 148–162). Dubuque, IA: McGraw-Hill.

Thaut, M. H.(1999b). *Training manual of Neurologic Music Therapy.* Ft. Collins, CO: Colorado State University, Center for Biomedical Research in Music.

Thaut, M. H. (2000). *A scientific model of music in therapy and medicine.* San Antonio, TX: IMR Press.

Thaut, M. H. (2001). *Neurologic Music Therapy.* Presentation at the annual meeting of the Midwestern Regional Chapter of the American Music Therapy Association, Kansas City, MO.

Thaut, M. H. (2005). *Rhythm, music, and the brain.* London, England: Taylor & Francis.

Thaut, M. H., & Davis, W. B. (1993). The influence of subject-selected versus experimenter-chosen music on affect, anxiety, and relaxation. *Journal of Music Therapy, 30,* 210–223.

Thaut, M. H., & de l'Etoile, S. K. (1993). The effects of music on mood state-dependent recall. *Journal of Music Therapy, 30,* 70–80.

Thaut, M. H., Leins, A. K., Rice, R. R., Argstatter, H., Kenyon, G. P., McIntosh, G. C., Bolay, H. V., & Fetter, M. (2007). Rhythmic auditory stimulation improves gait more than NDT/Bobath training in near-ambulatory patients early poststroke: A single-blind, randomized trial. *Neurorehabilitation and Neural Repair, 21*(5), 455–459.

Thaut, M. H., McIntosh, K. W., McIntosh, G. C., & Hoemberg, V. (2001). Auditory rhythmicity enhances movement and speech motor control in patients with Parkinson's disease. *Functional Neurology: New Trends in Adaptive and Behavioral Disorders, 16,* 163–172.

Thaut, M. H., McIntosh, G. C., Prassas, S. G., & Rice, R. R. (1992). Effect of rhythmic auditory cueing on temporal stride parameters and EMG patterns in normal gait. *Journal of Neurologic Rehabilitation, 6,* 185–190.

Thaut, M. H., McIntosh, G. C., & Rice, R. R. (1997). Rhythmic facilitation of gait training in hemiparetic stroke rehabilitation. *Journal of the Neurological Sciences, 151,* 207–212.

Thaut, M. H., Miltner, R., Lange, H. W., Hurt, C. P., & Hoemberg, V. (1999). Velocity modulation and rhythmic synchronization of gait in Huntington's disease. *Movement Disorders, 14*(5), 808–819.

Thaut, M. H., Peterson, D. A., & McIntosh G. C. (2005). Temporal entrainment of cognitive functions: Musical mnemonics induce brain plasticity and oscillatory synchrony in neural networks underlying memory. *Annals of the New York Academy of Sciences, 1060,* 243–254.

Thaut, M. H., Peterson, D. A., Sena, K. M., & McIntosh, G. C. (2008). Musical structure facilitates verbal learning in multiple sclerosis. *Music Perception, 25,* 325–330.

Thaut, M. H., Rathbun, J. A., & Miller, R. A. (1997). Music versus metronome timekeeper in a rhythmic motor task. *International Journal of Arts Medicine, 5*(1), 4–12.

Thaut, M. H., Schleiffers, S., & Davis, W. (1991). Analysis of EMG activity in biceps and triceps muscle in an upper extremity gross motor task under the influence of auditory rhythm. *Journal of Music Therapy, 28,* 64–88.

Thaut, M. H., Tian, B., & Azimi-Sadjadi, M. R. (1998). Rhythmic finger tapping to cosine-wave modulated metronome sequences: Evidence of subliminal entrainment. *Human Movement Science, 17,* 839–863.

Thiem, B., Green, D., Prassas, S., & Thaut, M. H. (1994). Left arm muscle activation and movement patterns in cellists employing a playing technique using rhythmic cuing. *Medical Problems of Performing Artists, 9,* 89–96.

Wallace, W. T. (1994). Memory for music: Effect of melody on recall of text. *Journal of Experimental Psychology, 20,* 1471–1485.

Recommended Additional Readings

Gardiner, J. (2005). Neurologic music therapy in cognitive rehabilitation. In M. H. Thaut (Ed.), *Rhythm, music, and the brain: Scientific foundation and clinical application* (pp. 179–201). New York: Routledge.

Molinari, M., Leggio, M. G., DeMartin, M., Cerasa, A., & Thaut, M. H. (2003). The neurobiology of rhythmic motor entrainment: A neurorehabilitation perspective. *Annals of the New York Academy of Sciences, 999,* 313–321.

Molinari, M., Leggio, M. G., & Thaut, M. H. (2007). The cerebellum and neural networks for rhythmic sensorimotor synchronization in the human brain. *Cerebellum, 6*(1), 18–23.

Peterson, D. A., & Thaut, M. H. (2007). Music increases frontal EEG coherence during verbal learning. *Neuroscience Letters, 412*(3), 217–221.

Sears, W. W. (1968). Processes in music therapy. In E. T. Gaston (Ed.), *Music in therapy* (pp. 30–44). New York: Macmillan.

Thaut, M. H. (1988). Rhythmic intervention techniques in music therapy with gross motor dysfunctions. *Arts in Psychotherapy, 15,* 127–137.

Thaut, M. H. (1989). Music therapy, affect modification, and therapeutic change: Towards an integrative model. *Music Therapy Perspectives, 7,* 55–62.

Thaut, M. H. (1997). Rhythmic auditory-motor facilitation of gait patterns in patients with Parkinson's disease. *Journal of Neurology, Neurosurgery and Psychiatry, 63*(1), 22–26.

Thaut, M. H. (1997). Rhythmic auditory stimulation in rehabilitation of movement disorders: A review of current research. In D. J. Schneck & J. K. Schneck (Eds.), *Music in human adaptation* (pp. 223–230). Blacksburg, VA: Virginia Polytechnic Institute and State University.

Thaut, M. H. (2002). Neuropsychological processes in music perception and their relevance in music therapy. In R. F. Unkefer & M. H. Thaut (Eds.), *Music therapy in the treatment of adults with mental disorders: Theoretical bases and clinical interventions* (pp. 2–32). St. Louis, MO: MMB Music.

Thaut, M. H. (2002). Physiological and motor responses to music stimuli. In R. F. Unkefer & M. H. Thaut (Eds.), *Music therapy in the treatment of adults with mental disorders: Theoretical bases and clinical interventions* (pp. 33–41). St. Louis, MO: MMB Music.

Thaut, M. H. (2003). Neural basis of rhythmic timing networks in the human brain. *Annals of the New York Academy of Sciences, 999,* 364–373.

Thaut, M. H. (2005). The future of music in therapy and medicine. *Annals of the New York Academy of Sciences, 1060,* 303–308.

Thaut, M. H. (2005). *Rhythm, music, and the brain.* London, England: Taylor & Francis.

Thaut, M. H., DeMartin, M., & Sanes, J. N. (2008). Brain networks for integrative rhythm formation. *PLoS One, 3*(5), e2312.

Thaut, M. H., Kenyon, G. P., Schauer, M. L., & McIntosh, G. C. (1999). Rhythmicity and brain function: Implication for therapy of movement disorders. *IEEE Engineering in Medicine and Biology, 18,* 101–108.

Chapter 11

The Biomedical Theory of Music Therapy

Dale B. Taylor

Introduction

For most of the general public, music is thought of as a form of entertainment, not as a treatment modality. For example, it is generally accepted that the product produced by a musician is music. However, it is difficult for most members of the general public to conceptualize a musician as one who provides treatment. When the profession began, music therapists did not claim to offer a "cure" for illnesses, but did offer music as a way of assisting with the emotional side of an illness or disability, as a means of improving quality of life for the patient, and as an aid in healing. When the inevitable question was asked concerning *how* music therapy works, one could offer a general definition of music therapy and anecdotes describing therapeutic benefits of musical participation. This explanation was followed closely by a description of the rigorous musical and clinical training required to become a music therapist. There was little scientific investigation to be reported that could "prove" that certain identifiable processes are at work creating treatment effects within the musical experience.

One response to the above dilemma was to classify music therapy within larger groups of therapeutic endeavors such as "activity therapy" or "adjunctive therapy." Another reaction was to identify certain music therapy procedures as belonging to other widely accepted intervention strategies such as "psychiatric music therapy" or "behavioral music therapy." No one term adequately explained the basis for music therapy itself as it is applied to all populations in all settings.

The Biomedical Theory of Music Therapy is not a set of procedures or a way of doing music therapy with any specified population group. It is instead a way of understanding and explaining why and how music is therapeutic in any intervention. This theoretical approach offers an independent conceptual basis for a definition of music therapy as well as for practice and research. It establishes the *brain* as the basic domain of treatment in all music therapy applications, and systematically and objectively defines music therapy interventions in terms that are applicable to the full range of client populations served. While there is continued discussion as to whether it is possible to objectify all musical responses scientifically, the fact remains that when each client's brain changes the way it governs behavior, music therapy then is able to show results.

It should be understood that the word *music* when used herein refers to a series of tones or combined tones, created with the intent of aesthetic expression and selected with full consideration of the specific musical background of individuals receiving music therapy treatment. It is recognized, however, that some research and clinical procedures utilize elements of music, such as rhythm or frequency, independently, rather than in combination with other musical elements.

History of the Biomedical Theory of Music Therapy

Since the earliest uses of music in society, man has observed that music is more than just a source of auditory enjoyment. The power of music to change moods, refocus attention, elicit emotions, express feelings, and socialize groups and individuals has been appreciated for centuries. The use of these influences in an organized professional discipline to affect therapeutic change is, however, a relatively recent development.

A review of the literature provides ample basis for development of a biomedical theory for the music therapy profession. For example, numerous published accounts contain clinical, anecdotal, and research findings relating the benefits of music in medical procedures. One such account written by Boxberger (1962) contains descriptions of the use of music to treat physical diseases, beginning as far back as primitive tribal culture. The long historical partnership between music and medicine from the time of the ancient Greeks up to the mid-1980s was reviewed by Pratt and Jones (1985). Pratt (1989) also provided a very useful history of music and medicine that focused in part on specific medical doctors who are associated with specific theories, research, and applications of music in medicine, and who have presided over worldwide organizations dedicated to investigating the relationship between music and medicine. In reviewing music and medicine in medieval Islamic and Judaic history, Sekeles (1988) provided a cross-cultural perspective that includes controlled research and spans various historical time periods. Also described are belief systems deeply rooted in religious philosophy that affected the medical latitude afforded to doctors.

Nineteenth century musical practices in hospitals in America are reflected in an article by Davis (1987). Selected articles are analyzed, which appeared in 19th century medical journals and dissertations between 1804 and 1899 and whose primary audience was physicians. An account by Taylor (1981) described musical practices in medicine during the first half of the 20th century and included experimental research, clinical applications, and college coursework covering music in medical-surgical hospitals and dentistry. Specific applications are described in which music was used as an integral part of treatment procedures in various departments of a general hospital such as pediatrics, surgery, orthopedics, and obstetrics. Standley (1986) analyzed a large number of reports, both published and unpublished, and constructed a profile of the subjects being studied, the types of research design being used, patterns of disseminating the information obtained, applications of music in medical procedures, and results of efforts to use music as therapy in the field of medicine. It was reported that of the 55 dependent variables analyzed in this study, 54 were found to have benefited more from the music condition than from the nonmusic condition regardless of whether the difference was significant. Such results tend to support the possibility of formulating a consistent and valid theory upon which to base further research as well as for interpreting currently available sets of data.

Biomedical theory has grown from a long history of research by investigators concerned with identifying biological components of music therapy. Although most prior attempts to explain music therapy did acknowledge physiological effects of music, the biological foundations of musical behavior had not been fully described, and music therapy had come to be known primarily for its applications to the cognitive and emotional problems of its clients. A large portion of the controlled research during the first half of the 20th century dealt with investigations into the physiological effects of music. Laboratory experiments done with both animals and humans demonstrated music-related changes in cardiac output, respiratory rate and volume, pulse rate, blood pressure, muscle tone, digestion, and body secretions (Taylor, 1981).

During the 1960s, research concerning the effectiveness of music as therapy focused on such behaviors as variations in heart rate, muscle potentials, galvanic skin response, pilomotor reflex, pain thresholds, changes in capillaries, postural changes, pupillary reflexes, and gastric motility (Sears & Sears, 1964). A treatise by Gaston (1964) described music as an aesthetic experience capable of enhancing uniquely human capacities and helping each person grow to his or her fullest potential as a human being. Much attention was given to the superior evolutionary development of man's highly complex brain and its hunger for sensory experience in the form of aesthetic stimuli such as music. The human species was portrayed as being distinguished by a greatly developed cerebrum consisting of billions of neurons, which enable complex speech patterns, abstract thinking, mathematical communication, and substantial amounts of nonverbal communication in various forms, including music.

During the decade of the 1980s, the fields of music and medicine experienced a re-awakening of their mutual interdependence. At a number of colleges and universities, partnerships were formed with medical hospitals in order to provide practical training of music therapists in various units such as maternity, obstetrics, oncology, rehabilitation, psychiatry, surgery, pediatrics, intensive care, cardiac care, cardiac rehabilitation, and general medical units. Practitioners were being prepared to use music in medical applications as well as to improve their knowledge of the biological and medical implications of music as therapy. Investigators such as Birbaumer (1983), Lee and Kella (1989), Hodges (1980), and Wilson (1989) began to study musical behavior in attempts to identify common factors in therapeutic, medical, educational, and aesthetic applications. These explorations placed great emphasis on the brain as the most comprehensive area of focus in studies of music behavior. In 1985, the *Wall Street Journal* published an article chronicling investigations of music/brain relationships (Stipp, 1985). It reported scientists as stating, "Music is a window on the brain," meaning that many brain functions could be studied effectively by using music.

Wilson (1988) and Manchester (1988) described implications of the biological processes involved in music making. Included are medical problems arising from music making as well as the use of music to treat physical problems. Wilson (1985) suggested that music and medicine are close to a rediscovery of their traditional bonds. The biomedical theory is intended to provide a practical foundation for professionals in both music and medicine to proceed with research and clinical applications of music in medical procedures. Upon hearing the biomedical theory presented, physicians have asserted repeatedly that knowledge of this theory would prompt the medical profession to listen and give the needed credibility to music therapy as a professional discipline.

The term *Biomedical Theory of Music Therapy* was first used in 1987 at the National Association for Music Therapy conference in San Francisco in this author's presentation titled "Therapeutic Musicians or Musical Physicians: The Future is at Stake," in which the need for the theory was identified. Once formulated, the first public presentation of the Biomedical Theory of Music Therapy was made at a research seminar held by the Commission on Music in Special Education, Music Therapy, and Music Medicine of the International Society for Music Education, held in Tallin, Estonia in 1990. The theory was first presented in the U.S. at the 1991 National Association for Music Therapy conference in San Diego.

Philosophical Orientation

The Biomedical Theory of Music Therapy is based upon a biological model of musical behavior. Its purpose is to provide a biomedical basis for interpreting receptive, expressive, and physiological behaviors of the human organism during musical participation. Its basic premise recognizes that there are specific neurophysiological structures and processes that must be activated in order for certain behavioral responses to occur. Therefore, any occurrence of those behaviors in response to musical stimuli must result from the effects of music on those same neurophysiological structures and processes. Knowledge of those musical effects enables their use in medical and other therapeutic applications.

The philosophical basis for the Biomedical Theory of Music Therapy rests on establishing the human brain as the basic domain of treatment and the primary focus for change in all music therapy applications. Scholars in the neurosciences have reported that "all human behavior is generated by the brain" (Hodges, 1980). This statement indicates that an enormous number of behavioral capabilities could be produced from at least 10 trillion known connections between neurons in the human brain. It also makes it incumbent upon students of any type of human behavior to study and become thoroughly familiar with the brain as it affects physical and cognitive behaviors. This certainly applies to anyone who studies music as therapy for clinical or educational applications. The basic biomedical theory holds that, because music has observable effects on human brain functioning, its effects can be used therapeutically. By emphasizing the human brain, it systematically and objectively defines music therapy interventions in terms that are applicable to the full range of client populations served.

In his 1964 treatise, Gaston explained that development of advanced human behaviors depends upon a process that begins with stimuli that are received by the sense organs, converted into sensation such as sound in the form of music, organized in accordance with the brain's own capacity for processing information, responded to in ways that are rational and individual rather than species-typical, and stored as memories to be recalled in response to future aesthetic stimuli. He asserted that a richer sensory environment leads to greater brain development. The brain, with its entire repertoire of coping potential, therefore depends upon the sense organs for its own development. The implication of his assertions clearly places sensory aesthetics at the forefront as a potential therapeutic modality for achieving enhanced human brain functioning. This point is extremely important since all music therapy goal-directed activity is aimed first and foremost at enhancing the functioning capacity of each client's brain.

Gaston reminded his readers that man is a biological unit and must relate to all else in accordance with biological principles. Such principles are reflected in the writings of noted aesthetic researcher Kate Hevner Mueller (1964), who explained pleasurable psychological responses to music in terms of electrochemical activity in the brain, which produces emotions as this activity is resolved. Two decades after Gaston assured his readers that the sense organs and the brain deserve our wonder, James (1984) proposed a sensory integration theory as a model for music therapy practice and research. *Sensory integration* refers to the process by which the nervous system receives and organizes tactile, proprioceptive, vestibular, olfactory, gustatory, visual, and auditory sensations. The degree to which individuals interact with their environment both before and after birth, therefore, is dependent upon their ability to process sensory information.

Sensory integration theorists believe that a major source of human adaptive capacity and learning is the ability to integrate stimuli from a variety of sensory sources. James asserted that the basic function of the central nervous system is to receive sensory information, screen and integrate meaningful stimuli, and respond motorically based on previous experience. This principle is *central* to an understanding of the Biomedical Theory of Music Therapy, as it is the therapist who elicits behavior by manipulating sensory input in order to control the information that the central nervous system works with in deciding how to respond.

Investigations of music/brain relationships provide the means for describing therapeutic influences of music in terms that explain objectively a basic domain, a single theoretical framework, which applies to *all* music therapy applications. The point of primary interest in the search for a universal domain of music therapy should be the brain. This conclusion is based on the fact that literally all of the work that music therapists do is primarily and ultimately aimed at changing the functions of specific biological structures of the human body. Such change *begins* with the brain, which must interpret any sound as "music" before that sound can exert a "musical" influence. For example, when treating psychiatric disorders, whether schizophrenic, borderline, bipolar, or any one of numerous other behavior disorders, the principal locus of the problem is in the client's *brain*. Also, with cognitive impairments in psychiatric or developmental disorders, it is the ability of the brain to process information and direct appropriate coping responses that determines the goals of the music therapist. In general hospital applications, one of the most widespread uses of music is to decrease pain perception by raising the threshold for pain stimuli reaching somatosensory portions of the patient's brain.

The ever-growing number of music therapists whose positions are in the long-term care industry find themselves working daily to combat the effects of Alzheimer's disease, arteriosclerosis, and cardiovascular diseases such as strokes, which have profound effects on the patient's brain. These brain diseases also have corresponding effects on other biological systems such as the circulatory and muscle systems. Clients whose disabilities are physical in nature receive music therapy intervention designed to improve physical functioning, a class of behavior which itself is totally dependent upon motivation and neurological control originating in the brain's limbic system and motor cortex. One of the more frequently seen physical disabilities, cerebral palsy, receives its name from its source, the brain. Intervention with clients having sensory disorders centers around finding ways to maximize the amount of environmental information accessible to the brain. Those exhibiting communication disorders such as aphasia receive music therapy treatment designed to utilize the functional plasticity of the human brain as it reassigns tasks to compensate for processing and motor planning capabilities lost due to damage in specialized speech centers. Because biomedical theory focuses so directly on the brain, it is necessary that the practitioner has some familiarity with basic neurophysiology, brain pathology, and perhaps neuromusicology, psychomusicology, neuroimmunology, neurochemistry, and physiological psychology.

Harvey (1987) reviewed research in the fields of music and medicine that point to a convergence of the two fields. He cited numerous clinical research studies indicating that music does have a predictable effect on human behavior during medical procedures. An institute for further study of the music–mind–medicine relationship was proposed based, in part, on the following three assumptions, which parallel basic tenets of the Biomedical Theory of Music Therapy:

1. The center of control for the human organism is the brain.
2. Music is processed by the brain and through the brain, after which it can then affect us in many ways.
3. Music can have a positive effect upon both neural functions and hormonal activity and, as such, can facilitate the healthy functioning of the body's own immune and regenerative processes. (Harvey, 1987, pp. 73–74)

By viewing music therapy from the perspective of brain functioning, it should be no longer necessary to refer to the therapeutic influences of music as magical, mystical, or unexplainable. An important goal in formulating the biomedical theory is to demystify music as therapy by providing information needed to understand neurophysiological responses to music that take place in tangible and familiar structures of the human organism. An understanding of the Biomedical Theory of Music Therapy will provide both a theoretical framework within which to make informed decisions concerning selection and application of music in medicine, as well as a philosophical foundation for further research.

Description of the Biomedical Theory of Music Therapy

The biomedical theory has an eclectic focus and is not one approach to be placed beside or above any others. Rather, it is a way of understanding and explaining what is actually taking place when any music therapy intervention is utilized. Three fundamental preliminary assumptions form a conceptual core around which the biomedical music therapist plans clinical interventions utilizing musical influences: (a) music affects each human being only because of the neurophysiological structures that each person possesses for receiving and responding to sound in the form of music; (b) participation in music, whether receptive or expressive in nature, activates a wide range of specific and identifiable physiological and neuropsychological processes in the human body; and (c) musically activated neurophysiological responses are observable, measurable, and predictable, thus affording selection of music activities having predetermined positive effects on patients during medical procedures.

These three assumptions, as well as all applications of music as therapy, depend upon the same neurophysiological process: Once sensory stimuli in the form of musical sounds are received in the ear, they activate use of the auditory tract, enter the central nervous system via the medulla, and, after passing through the thalamus, they are processed in the cerebral cortex. The brain develops its capacities in part because sense organs, such as the ears, which accomplish transduction of sound waves, transmit the energy that generates brain development. The brain decodes and converts information and experience entering in the form of nerve impulses into sensations. It subsequently organizes and identifies stimuli, selects and directs reactions, stores information about the whole process, and recalls it as needed. By indulging in these operations, the brain develops its capacity for rationality, verbal and nonverbal communication, quantitative and qualitative computation, abstract thinking, and control of motor behavior. Music facilitates this development by involving nearly all areas of the brain in perceiving and responding to musical stimuli during both receptive and expressive participation. Cromie (2001) reported that studies done of people with brain damage, and brain scans of people taken during music listening, show that music perception results from the neural exchange of activity in both hemispheres. Some neural circuits in the brain respond specifically to music but also process other forms of sound. The example given was that the area of the brain that processes perfect pitch also is active in perception of speech. In processing various musical elements, the right hemisphere was identified as essential for pitch perception as well as for some characteristics of harmony, melody, timbre, and rhythm. The left hemisphere is more accurate in dealing with rapid frequency and intensity changes in music as well as in words. However, both hemispheres are needed for adequate perception of rhythm, such as in determining the difference between three-quarter and four-quarter metric patterns. The frontal cortex of the brain, where working memory is stored, also is involved in perception of rhythm and melody.

The Biomedical Theory of Music Therapy itself states that "music influences human behavior by affecting the brain and subsequently other bodily structures in ways that are observable, identifiable, measurable, and predictable, thereby providing the necessary foundation for its use in treatment procedures." This basic principle applies to the effects of music on pain, emotion, communication skills, motor activity, stress, and cognition. biomedical theory explains that because all sound stimuli perceived in the primary auditory cortex also have a secondary effect on all parts of the brain, sound as music affects pain perception through its ability to stimulate nerves in the midbrain. This results in inhibition of pain sensations attempting to enter the central nervous system following reception by sensors in the peripheral nervous system. Another biologically based explanation has enlisted the arousal functions of the reticular activating system (RAS). It says that receptive musical audiation depresses awareness of pain indirectly by causing the reticular activating system to arouse the brain to focus on music instead of on pain sensations (Cook, 1981). However, it has not been determined why music would be chosen over the many other stimuli available to the RAS at any given time. Still, the presence of music has been determined to produce analgesia—a reduction in sensitivity to pain. One application of biomedical theory is to explain pain reduction through music. Such an explanation is contained in the following section on Applications of the Biomedical Theory of Music Therapy.

Another basic tenet of biomedical theory holds that because the final relay station in the normal auditory pathway is in the thalamus, this allows music to immediately affect the hypothalamus, which works closely with the limbic system in controlling emotional behavior. Musically stimulated positive emotional responses may thereby inhibit negative reactions that can delay or otherwise interfere with the treatment or recovery process. The ability of music to elicit emotional responses is used as a therapeutic tool in many applications.

The third biomedical principle emphasizes the importance of the brain in all endeavors involving bodily movement and, consequently, its importance in rehabilitation of motor functions in patients. It states that active participation in expressive musical activities provides structured movement behaviors necessary for maintenance or recovery of physical function, and for development of the skills necessary for interpersonal communication. Selection of music activities to utilize the interdependence of the brain and muscles must be based on a thorough understanding of normal neuromuscular functioning within the human body. An important part of this principle involves knowledge of the language centers in the human brain and the behavioral correlates associated with their pathologies. Also important is an understanding of the principle of "functional neuroplasticity," in which the brain takes tasks that would be assigned to damaged cerebral tissue and performs those tasks in undamaged cranial areas. The use of music to enhance this process explains musically facilitated skill recovery. A system has been developed for applying this principle to aphasia treatment and is cited in the following section.

Historically, the most widely accepted application of music as a therapeutic agent is its use as a calming agent to combat anxiety, tension, and stress. The need to appropriately manage stress is easily understood through the many widely recognized effects of excess stress on human health and behavior. These effects include the development of physical problems such as hypertension, ulcers, skin disorders, headaches, arteriosclerosis, reproductive dysfunctions, coronary disease, respiratory ailments, and changes in lymphocyte levels that increase the risk of cancer. Also associated with anxiety and stress are fluid retention, obesity, psychosomatic symptoms, and increased rates of depression and suicide (Hanser, 1985). Perhaps because of the many physiological changes that attend these states, anxiety has come to be identified by its numerous associated physiological changes, including such parameters as heart rate, blood pressure, galvanic skin response, and electromyographic and electroencephalographic responses. Individuals cope with anxiety or stress by attempting to confront or remove the stress-provoking source or by managing it through relaxation.

Use of music to induce relaxation reflects the fourth principle of the Biomedical Theory of Music Therapy. It states that music has a direct effect on specific physiological processes whose functional variations are indicators of anxiety, tension, or stress. To understand the effects of music on the physiology of anxiety and stress, it is necessary to more closely examine parts of the limbic system and their relationship to hormonal secretions from the endocrine glands. Studies show that the central nucleus of the amygdala sends projections to parts of the brain that react to aversive stimuli. These include portions of the lower brain stem that are involved in controlling the autonomic nervous system and a nucleus in the hypothalamus whose activity results in the secretion of stress-related hormones. When the perception of an aversive situation results in stimulation of the central nucleus of the amygdala, there are resulting increases in heart rate and blood pressure, which contribute to the awareness of physiological changes during anxiety. Carlson (1992) has shown that gastric ulcers may be produced if stimulation is long-term. It follows, therefore, that the autonomic responses controlled by the central nucleus of the amygdala can be causally related to the harmful effects of long-term stress, such as circulatory, coronary, and gastric problems.

The amygdala also is involved in organizing behavioral responses to emotions such as anger and its behavioral correlate, aggression. It also mediates fear reactions, which result in defensive responses. It is important to consider that both anger and fear are object-related emotions. An individual feels anger at, and fear of, something or someone. Like fear, anxiety also is an emotional response to specific internal and external stimuli. It contains all of the same elements of the fear emotion, except it is not directed toward immediate action or thought that would remove the effect of the stimulus (Birbaumer, 1983). When responses to the object of one's anger, fear, or anxiety continue over an extended period of time without resolution or reduction, the neurophysiological responses that constitute these feelings also persist, often with serious harmful effects, such as high blood pressure due to prolonged stimulation of the central nucleus of the amygdala (Carlson, 1992).

The fifth basic principle addressed in biomedical theory describes the role of music in facilitating use and development of cognitive capabilities in the human brain. Cognition in any endeavor involves the brain in perception or recall of information and stimuli, processing of that data, and selection and execution of a response. Musical perception and participation require the brain to organize incoming stimuli and to plan and execute corresponding behavior, thereby enhancing perceptual ability, cognitive processing, and interactive response capability. Because musical and other experiences are processed in areas located throughout the brain, such experience, especially in childhood, may have positive effects on developing capabilities that contribute to development of a range of cognitive skills. This was essentially the theory tested by Chan, Cheung, and Ho (2003), who sought to determine whether the impact of early life experience on cognitive functions is predictable if effects of that experience on neuroanatomy can be determined. They cited recent work indicating that verbal memory is mediated primarily in the left temporal lobe, while visual memory is processed in the right temporal lobe. Based on findings of left temporal enlargement among musicians, they then tested the effects of experience in music training on improvement in children's verbal and visual memory. They hypothesized that if neuroanatomical change accompanies changes in localized cognitive function, then subjects with music training should do better on verbal memory tasks but not visual memory, since their left temporal lobe has been shown to be better developed. Results revealed that children with music training did show better verbal but not visual memory than those without musical experience. When followed up 1 year later, those who had begun or continued formal music training demonstrated significant improvement in verbal memory, whereas children who did not continue music showed no improvement. The authors concluded that music training may systematically affect memory processing in accordance with neuroanatomical alterations in the left temporal lobe.

Clinical Applications of the Biomedical Theory of Music Therapy

Biomedical theory gains part of its applicability through its explanation of how music results in decreased pain awareness in the many examples of the use of music to decrease overt pain responses, reduce pain sensations, and decrease amounts of anesthetic or analgesic medication needed both during and following surgical and obstetrical procedures. Pain generally results from events that cause damage to skin and other kinds of tissue. Hence, it has a positive role in notifying the brain that something has gone wrong in an area of the body. Free nerve endings are the receptors for painful stimuli and are found in skin, in membranes covering muscles, in tissue lining the joints, and in the body of muscles. An injury results in rupture of a capillary and tissue cells, thereby stimulating mast cells to release *bradykinin*, a molecule that causes the free nerve endings to fire, sending pain impulses via peripheral nerves toward the central nervous system. Axons carrying pain impulses enter the central nervous system through dorsal root ganglia in the dorsal horn of the spinal cord, where they form synapses with other neurons. The axons from this next relay of neurons cross to the contralateral side of the spinal cord and ascend to the ventral posterior nuclei of the thalamus, which, in turn, project axons to the primary somatosensory cortex located behind the central sulcus in the human brain (Carlson, 1992; Mader, 1995).

It is generally believed among investigators that peptide neurotransmitters are active in the control of sensitivity to pain. Serotonin, a monoamine transmitter, is released at most synapses and participates in the regulation of pain by producing inhibitory postsynaptic potentials. Since the early 1970s, investigators have known that pain perception can be modified by a variety of environmental stimuli. Volumes of reports from medical and dental uses of music have established that music is one of the more reliable of these environmental stimuli. By activating analgesia-producing neural circuits, these stimuli induce the release of endogenous opiates in the brain, which then stimulate opiate receptors on neurons in the periaqueductal gray matter of the thalamus. Connections from the periaqueductal gray matter activate neurons located in the nucleus raphe magnus of the medulla. These neurons then send axons to the gray matter of the dorsal horn of the spinal cord, where their function is to inhibit the activity of neurons bringing pain information into the CNS for transmission to the brain. There is ample literature affirming that music has been found to enhance endorphin production (Scarantino, 1987). There also are many studies reporting success in applying music for analgesia. Real-time measurements of pain stimuli in surgery, obstetrics, oncology, burn centers, and pain clinics should show decreases with application of musical stimuli.

Another clinical application of the Biomedical Theory of Music Therapy is its use in explaining the basis of the observed effect of music in reducing anxiety and enhancing immune system function, which can be decreased during periods of stress. A grasp of this explanation requires some understanding of the physiology of anxiety and stress. Stress refers to the physiological reaction caused by the continuous perception of threatening situations. The perception of such threats generates a sustained stress reaction in which the adrenal glands secrete epinephrine, which affects glucose metabolism; norepinephrine, which increases heart output and blood pressure; and steroid stress hormones, such as cortisol. Research has shown, however, that music can significantly reduce pulse rate and plasma levels of epinephrine, norepinephrine, and cortisol in patients undergoing medical and dental procedures (Spintge & Droh, 1987).

Cortisol is a *glucocorticoid* that serves to conserve blood glucose by profoundly affecting glucose metabolism, helping break down protein and converting it to glucose, and increasing blood flow. Sustained stress results in prolonged secretion of glucocorticoids with long-term effects such as high blood pressure, increased risk of heart attacks and strokes, steroid diabetes, infertility, inhibition of the inflammatory response, destruction of neurons in parts of the hippocampus, and suppression of the immune system by interfering with the ability of white blood cells to combat infections. In addition to extended situations that elicit stress reactions, immediate occurrences can cause an increase in pituitary ACTH (adrenocorticotropic hormone) that controls the secretion of cortisol by the adrenal cortex. The largest hormonal increases occur with presentation of aversive events that are either completely unpredictable or completely predictable (Birbaumer, 1983).

A biomedical application would include the use of music to decrease neuronal signals from the amygdala to the hypothalamus, which in turn controls pituitary output of ACTH. Reductions in ACTH will result in reduced production of cortisol and other glucocorticoids, thus allowing the immune system freedom to be effective in combating infections. Use of music to achieve physical and emotional relaxation is also important in hemodialysis, surgery, and pediatrics.

A biomedically prepared music therapist working in a hospital or psychiatric setting where emotional instability is a major impediment to progress would work to help the client regain control of his or her emotions through reconditioning the conditioned emotional responses controlled by the amygdala. An additional objective would be to achieve increased serotonin levels in the brain. Such levels have been found to be below normal in depressed clients as well as those with eating disorders. Application of the biomedical theory requires that the practitioner be familiar with the roles played by various portions of the limbic system, including the amygdala, orbitofrontal cortex, hippocampal formation, and a closely related structure known as the cingulate gyrus. Changes in the behaviors handled by these structures require that the music therapist accomplish music-related stimulation of those structures. Also, it may not be enough to know simply how to reinforce target behaviors in therapy. It becomes important to be able to identify the neuropsychological and biochemical aspects of brain reinforcement brought about by musical stimuli.

A clinical explanation reflecting biomedical theory in psychiatry can be found in the work of Montello (1999), who uses a Psychoanalytic Music Therapy approach to treat adults who have been traumatized as children. Psychoanalytic techniques are designed to activate inborn individualized musicality and to use creative expression to heal the splits in a personality shattered by abuse. Montello points out that music bypasses the defenses of the brain's higher cortical functions and directly affects emotional processing in the limbic system. Even more specifically, she acknowledges the use of music to stimulate the right side of the brain to involve imagination and feelings. She also indicates how traumatized clients are not aware of how their overcharged nervous systems distort natural life rhythms that accompany life experiences. So much energy is expended on years of repressed or unexpressed rage and fear, that this internal battle "can take its toll on the nervous system, the endocrine system, and, in turn, the immune system" (p. 77), which can leave one susceptible to viruses, feeling exhausted, and unable to live life according to natural rhythms.

An application of the Biomedical Theory of Music Therapy that has received substantial attention is its use in treating aphasic disorders. Research using real-time brain scans shows where the brain is most active during specific receptive musical tasks. Because the speech and language centers, whose damage leads to aphasia, are found in the left cranial hemisphere, and because scans during music show the brain to be quite active in both hemispheres, a neuroanatomical model has been developed for using music to help the brain regain lost functions by redeveloping those skills in a different cranial location (Taylor, 1989). Using carefully sequenced musical experiences, aphasic clients are able to regain expressive or receptive language skills lost due to brain damage.

Although not reversible with current medical interventions, patients exhibiting Alzheimer's dementia and arteriosclerosis have been shown to exhibit cognitive skills involving memory, social skills, and physical coordination during musical participation that are not seen during nonmusical activity. An understanding of the biology of these diseases will make it clear to the therapist that they are brain disorders. Their treatment should, therefore, be approached from the standpoint of maximizing residual brain functions, some of which may be functional although not exhibited outside of musical interventions.

A treatment area that can be better understood through application of biomedical theory involves re-activation of cognitive operations in coma patients. Musical stimuli have been shown to arouse the brains of some patients sufficiently to reactivate their perceptual, processing, and response capabilities to observable levels (Boyle, 1989). Research studies of electrical responses in the brain also show measurable arousal patterns in response to music (Barber, McKenzie, & Helme, 1997). Differences were found in brain electrical activation between music and resting state conditions in all bandwidths and at all scalp regions having electrode locations. The observed activation patterns clearly demonstrate that musical perception activates neurological processes and thereby changes neural impulse patterning in the brain.

Related Research

The research basis for the Biomedical Theory of Music Therapy is extensive and expanding. A foundation for such research has been established through historical research completed by Boxberger (1962), Davis (1987), Pratt (1989), and Taylor (1981). Medical doctors also have been major participants in the building of a scientific relationship between music and biology as a basis for music as therapy. Notable among these are Lee and Kella (1989), Spintge and Droh (1987), Oyama, Hatano, et al. (1983), Oyama, Sato, Kudo, Spintge, and Droh (1983), Miluk-Kolasa (1993), Tanioka et al. (1985), Halpaap, Spintge, Droh, Kummert, and Kogel (1985), and Wilson (1989). Goff, a retired dental surgeon, teamed with Pratt and Madrigal (1997) to study musical effects during dental procedures. While most music therapists have not ventured into investigations of the effects of music on biological responses, notable among the participants in such studies are Thaut, Brown, Benjamin, and Cooke (1994), Staum (1983), and Taylor (1973), all of whom completed studies that involved measurement of physiological variables during musical experience.

Many music therapy investigators are studying musical applications in general hospital units to determine their effects on patients undergoing medical procedures. Among these are Standley (1999), Caine (1991), and Whipple (2000), who studied the effects of music in the Neonatal Intensive Care Unit; Robb (2000), Weber, Nuessler, and Wilmanns (1997), Kennelly (2001), Daveson (2001), and Waldon (2001), who studied oncology patients; Curtis (1986), who studied pain awareness in terminally ill patients; Clark, McCorkle, and Williams (1981), Hanser, Larson, and O'Connell (1983), and Browning (2001), who studied mothers during childbirth; Baker (2001), who studied posttraumatic amnesia patients; Boyle (1989), who studied coma patients; Rudenberg and Christenberry (1993) and Christenberry (1979), who looked at music therapy applications with burn patients; and Pratt (1999), Mandel (1988), Chetta (1981), and Gibbons and McDougal (1987), who are among those who reported on music during surgery.

Other investigators from the fields of music, music education, medicine, and psychology are contributing greatly to the biomedical foundations of music as therapy. They include work by Coleman, Pratt, Stoddard, Gerstmann, and Hans-Henning (1997) in the premature infant ICU;

Barber, McKenzie, and Helme (1997), Panksepp and Bekkedal (1997), and Altenmuller, Gruhn, Parlitz, and Kahrs (1997), who measured EEG changes resulting from musical experience; and Cromie (2001), who reported observations of brain scans taken during music listening. Other investigators such as Babic (1993) and Woodward (1992) have focused on developing knowledge of prenatal musical perception and sound cognition. Much of this research is in disciplines outside of music therapy and involves direct investigation of the effects of music as a variable.

Conclusion

Although there is an expanding body of research showing positive therapeutic effects of music independent of other influences, the field of music therapy previously has not been able to incorporate these findings into an integrated independent philosophy of music therapy that would explain why music is therapeutic. By adopting an interdisciplinary view of the theoretical basis for music therapy, it is possible to discover countless correlates between the effects of music and findings from other fields about the realities of human behavior. Much of the research in other disciplines involves direct investigation of the effects of music as a variable. What emerges from such an interdisciplinary overview is the realization that the vast majority of those studies involve attempts to understand the workings of the human brain. Because the brain is central to music and to nearly all other observable human behavior, it therefore must be a major focus of any comprehensive theory of music therapy. The advantage is that brain functions can be studied and reported scientifically instead of continuing to rely on claims of the "magical" or "mystical" power of music.

Modern music therapists are rediscovering music as therapy through investigations of its direct effects on the human nervous system. Medical doctors also have been major participants in the building of a scientific relationship between music and neurology that has established the brain as the important link between musical effects and human responses. In his discussion of the biology of music, Wilson (1989) mentions the role of the basal ganglia in task learning and cites studies showing that responses in the dentate nucleus of the cerebellum preceded activation of neurons in the precentral (motor) cortex by as much as 33 msec. Wilson went on to predict a much closer relationship between brain science and music.

Through the new and growing relationship between music and neurology, a rediscovery of the function of music as therapy has taken place. Investigators and practitioners are realizing that the therapeutic role of music in clinical applications is much broader and more important than previously thought. Its effects are much more specific, describable, and predictable than past therapists dared claim. Future therapists who are well versed in biomedical theory and who remain current with recent findings will be able to describe in detail musical effects that have been previously considered mystical and incapable of being analyzed or explained. The new knowledge, when viewed collectively, leads to a redefinition of music therapy as a discipline with the human brain as its central focus. The biomedical definition states that "Music therapy is the enhancement of human capabilities through the planned use of musical influences on brain functioning."

The Biomedical Theory of Music Therapy provides a unifying conceptual framework for many of the various theoretical positions and clinical modalities existing within music therapy.

Music therapists who practice and who describe their practice in relation to biomedical theory are becoming recognized as medical specialists functioning as equals with their professional peers. They are able to explain music therapy using terminology and functional parameters familiar to other health and medical practitioners and are able to be understood on the same medically sound basis as other disciplines. Professional credentialing requirements should include assessment techniques that measure knowledge of neurophysiological parameters that respond to music, and the ability to bring about positive changes in those parameters using musical experiences.

Substantial progress has been made in building a research base specific to biomedical effects of music. Donald Hodges, Director of the Institute for Music Research, and Terry Mikiten, Associate Dean of the Graduate School of Biomedical Sciences, both of the University of Texas at San Antonio, have cited seven benefits of increased knowledge about relationships between music, the brain, and human behavior. In their presentation to a 1994 conference of the International Society for Music in Medicine, they predicted: (a) better understanding and appreciation of the role of music in human life; (b) greater recognition that music is not just a diversion, but has a significant impact on human physiology and psychology; (c) an awareness that music can have a significant positive or negative effect on human behavior; (d) increased efficiency in educating people musically; (e) improvements in preparing performing musicians and in dealing with their injuries; (f) increased efficiency in using music to improve the quality of life for handicapped individuals; and (g) expanded use of music as treatment for medical and other widely varied clinical conditions such as childbirth, brain injury, or chronic pain. The Biomedical Theory of Music Therapy offers conclusions that are based on substantial amounts of interdisciplinary research data. It offers a framework within which to draw coordinated conclusions from disparate sources based on the behavior of human parameters that can be understood by both music therapists and professional colleagues in other clinical disciplines.

The reader should note, as exemplified by Montello (1999), that the addition of the brain to any approach to explaining musical influence requires absolutely *no* mention of the "Biomedical Theory of Music Therapy" as a theoretical position. It also should be noted that, although experience and feedback from early use of the theory have consistently demonstrated that a biomedically based explanation of music therapy can bring noticeable benefits to the profession, the reader should *not* interpret this to mean that this theory should replace or subsume any current or previous theoretical approach to explaining this discipline. Rather, it is believed that this theoretical approach can support all approaches to music therapy intervention and that all should continue to be practiced and developed by their various practitioners and advocates.

References

Altenmuller, E., Gruhn, W., Parlitz, D., & Kahrs, J. (1997). Music learning produces changes in brain activation patterns: A longitudinal DC-EEG study. *International Journal of Arts Medicine, 5*(1), 28–33.

Babic, Z. (1993). Towards a linguistic framework of prenatal language stimulation. In T. Blum (Ed.), *Prenatal perception, learning and bonding* (pp. 361–386). Hong Kong: Leanardo.

Baker, F. (2001). The effects of live, taped, and no music on people experiencing posttraumatic amnesia. *Journal of Music Therapy, 38,* 170–192.

Barber, B., McKenzie, S., & Helme, R. (1997). A study of brain electrical responses to music using quantitative electroencephalography (QEEG). *International Journal of Arts Medicine, 5*(2), 12–21.

Birbaumer, N. (1983). The psychophysiology of anxiety. In R. Spintge & R. Droh (Eds.), *Anxiety, pain and music in anesthesia* (pp. 23–30). Basel, Germany: Editiones Roches.

Boxberger, R. (1962). Historical bases for the use of music in therapy. In E. Schneider (Ed.), *Music therapy 1961* (pp. 125–166). Lawrence, KS: National Association for Music Therapy.

Boyle, M. E. (1989). Comatose and head injured patients: Applications for music in treatment. In M. H. M. Lee (Ed.), *Rehabilitation, music and human well-being* (pp. 137–148). St. Louis: MMB Music.

Browning, C. A. (2001). Music therapy in childbirth: Research in practice. *Music Therapy Perspectives, 19*(2), 74–81.

Caine, J. (1991). The effects of music on the selected stress behaviors, weight, caloric and formula intake, and length of hospital stay of premature and low birth weight neonates in a newborn intensive care unit. *Journal of Music Therapy, 28,* 180–192.

Carlson, N. R. (1992). *Foundations of physiological psychology.* Boston: Allyn & Bacon.

Chan, A., Cheung, M., & Ho, Y. (2003). Music training improves verbal but not visual memory: Cross-sectional and longitudinal explorations in children. *Neuropsychology, 17*(3), 439–450.

Chetta, H. D. (1981). The effect of music and desensitization on preoperative anxiety in children. *Journal of Music Therapy, 18,* 74–87.

Christenberry, E. B. (1979). The use of music therapy with burn patients. *Journal of Music Therapy, 16,* 138–148.

Clark, M., McCorkle, R., & Williams, S. (1981). Music therapy-assisted labor and delivery. *Journal of Music Therapy, 18,* 88–100.

Coleman, J. M., Pratt, R. R., Stoddard, R. A., Gerstmann, D. R., & Hans-Henning, A. (1997). The effects of the male and female singing and speaking voices on selected physiological and behavioral measures of premature infants in the intensive care unit. *International Journal of Arts Medicine, 5*(2), 4–11.

Cook, J. D. (1981). The therapeutic use of music: A literature review. *Nursing Forum, 20,* 252–266.

Cromie, W. (2001). Music on the brain: Researchers explore the biology of music. *Harvard University Gazette.* Retrieved from http://www.hno.harvard.edu/gazette/2001/03.22/04-music.html

Curtis, S. (1986). The effect of music on pain relief and relaxation of the terminally ill. *Journal of Music Therapy, 23,* 10–24.

Daveson, B. A. (2001). Music therapy and childhood cancer: Goals, methods, patient choice and control during diagnosis, intensive treatment, transplant and palliative care. *Music Therapy Perspectives, 19*(2), 114–120.

Davis, W. (1987). Music therapy in 19th century America. *Journal of Music Therapy, 24,* 76–87.

Gaston, E. T. (1964). The aesthetic experience and biological man. *Journal of Music Therapy, 1,* 1–7.

Gibbons, A. C., & McDougal, D. L. (1987). Music therapy in medical technology: Organ transplants. In R. Pratt (Ed.), *The Fourth International Symposium on Music: Rehabilitation and human well-being* (pp. 61–72). Basel, Germany: Editiones Roches.

Goff, L. C., Pratt, R. R., & Madrigal, J. L. (1997). Music listening and S-IgA levels in patients undergoing dental procedure. *International Journal of Arts Medicine, 5*(2), 22–26.

Halpaap, B., Spintge, R., Droh, R., Kummert, W., & Kogel, W. (1985). Anxiolytic music in obstetrics. In R. Spintge & R. Droh (Eds.), *Music in medicine* (pp. 145–154). Basel, Germany: Editiones Roches.

Hanser, S., Larson, S., & O'Connell, A. (1983). The effect of music on relaxation of expectant mothers during labor. *Journal of Music Therapy, 20,* 50–58.

Hanser, S. B. (1985). Music therapy and stress reduction research. *Journal of Music Therapy, 22,* 193–206.

Harvey, A. W. (1987). Utilizing music as a tool for healing. In R. Pratt (Ed.), *The Fourth International Symposium on Music: Rehabilitation and human well-being* (pp. 73–87). Basel, Germany: Editiones Roches.

Hodges, D. A. (1980). Neurophysiology and human hearing. In D. Hodges (Ed.), *Handbook of music psychology* (p. 195). Dubuque, IA: Kendall/Hunt.

James, M. R. (1984). Sensory integration: A theory for therapy and research. *Journal of Music Therapy, 21,* 79–88.

Kennelly, J. (2001). Music therapy in the bone marrow transplant unit: Providing emotional support during adolescence. *Music Therapy Perspectives, 19*(2), 104–108.

Lee, M. H. M., & Kella, J. J. (1989). Computerized thermography and other technological aids in the diagnosis of musicians' neuromuscular disorders. In M. H. M. Lee (Ed.), *Rehabilitation, music and human well-being* (pp. 37–56). St. Louis, MO: MMB Music.

Mader, S. S. (1995). *Human biology.* Dubuque, IA: Wm. C. Brown.

Manchester, R. A. (1988). Medical aspects of music development. *Psychomusicology, 7,* 147–152.

Mandel, S. E. (1988). Music therapy: A personal peri-surgical experience. *Music Therapy Perspectives, 5,* 109–110.

Miluk-Kolasa, B. (1993). *Effects of listening to music on selected physiological variables and anxiety level in pre-surgical patients.* Unpublished doctoral dissertation, Medical University of Warsaw, Poland.

Montello, L. (1999). A psychoanalytic music therapy approach to treating adults traumatized as children. *Music Therapy Perspectives, 16,* 74–81.

Mueller, K. H. (1964). The aesthetic experience and psychological man. *Journal of Music Therapy, 1*(1), 8–10.

Oyama, T., Hatano, K., Sato, Y., Kudo, T., Spintge, R., & Droh, R. (1983). Endocrine effect of anxiolytic music in dental patients. In R. Spintge & R. Droh (Eds.), *Anxiety, pain and music in anesthesia* (pp. 143–146). Basel, Germany: Editiones Roches.

Oyama, T., Sato, Y., Kudo, T., Spintge, R., & Droh, R. (1983). Effect of anxiolytic music on endocrine function in surgical patients. In R. Spintge & R. Droh (Eds.), *Anxiety, pain and music in anesthesia* (pp. 147–152). Basel, Germany: Editiones Roches.

Panksepp, J., & Bekkedal, M. Y. V. (1997). The affective cerebral consequence of music: Happy vs. sad effects on the EEG and clinical implications. *International Journal of Arts Medicine, 5*(1), 18–27.

Pratt, R. R. (1989). A brief history of music and medicine. In M. H. M. Lee (Ed.), *Rehabilitation, music and human well-being* (pp. 1–12). St. Louis, MO: MMB Music.

Pratt, R. R. (1999). Listening to music during surgery: A program of intermountain health. *International Journal of Arts Medicine, 6*(1), 21–30.

Pratt, R. R., & Jones, R. W. (1985). Music and medicine: A partnership in history. In R. Spintge & R. Droh (Eds.), *Music in medicine* (pp. 307–318). Basel, Germany: Editiones Roches.

Robb, S. L. (2000). The effect of therapeutic music interventions on the behavior of hospitalized children in isolation: Developing a contextual support model of music therapy. *Journal of Music Therapy, 37,* 118–146.

Rudenberg, M. T., & Christenberry, A. R. (1993). Promoting psychological adjustment in pediatric burn patients through music therapy and child life therapy. In R. Pratt (Ed.), *Music therapy and music education for the handicapped* (pp. 164–165). St. Louis, MO: MMB Music.

Scarantino, B. A. (1987). *Music power.* New York: Dodd, Mead.

Sears, M. L., & Sears, W. W. (1964). Abstracts of research in music therapy. *Journal of Music Therapy, 1,* 33–60.

Sekeles, C. (1988). Convergent points between music and medicine as reflected in a number of examples in medieval Islamic and Judaic history. *Journal of the International Association of Music for the Handicapped, 3,* 14–24.

Spintge, R., & Droh, R. (1987). Effects of anxiolytic music on plasma levels of stress hormones in different medical specialties. In R. Pratt (Ed.), *The Fourth International Symposium on Music: Rehabilitation and human well-being* (pp. 88–101). Lanham, MD: University Press of America.

Standley, J. M. (1986). Music research in medical/dental treatment: Meta-analysis and clinical applications. *Journal of Music Therapy, 23,* 56–122.

Standley, J. M. (1999). Music therapy in the NICU: Pacifier-activated lullabies (PAL) for reinforcement of nonnutritive sucking. *International Journal of Arts Medicine, 6*(2), 17–21.

Staum, M. J. (1983). Music and rhythmic stimuli in the rehabilitation of gait disorders. *Journal of Music Therapy, 20,* 69–87.

Stipp, D. (1985, August 30). What happens when music meets the brain? *Wall Street Journal,* p. 1.

Tanioka, F., Takazawa, T., Kamata, S., Kudo, M., Matsuki, A., & Oyama, T. (1985). Hormonal effect of anxiolytic music in patients during surgical operations under epidural anesthesia. In R. Spintge & R. Droh (Eds.), *Music in medicine* (pp. 285–290). Basel, Germany: Editiones Roches.

Taylor, D. B. (1973). Subject responses to precategorized stimulative and sedative music. *Journal of Music Therapy, 10,* 86–94.

Taylor, D. B. (1981). Music in general hospital treatment from 1900–1950. *Journal of Music Therapy, 18,* 62–73.

Taylor, D. B. (1987). *Therapeutic musicians or musical physicians: The future is at stake.* Paper presented at the annual meeting of the National Association for Music Therapy, San Francisco.

Taylor, D. B. (1989). A neuroanatomical model for the use of music in the remediation of aphasic disorders. In M. Lee (Ed.), *Rehabilitation, music and human well-being* (pp. 168–178). St. Louis, MO: MMB Music.

Taylor, D. B. (1990). *A biomedical theory of music therapy and its implications for training and research.* Paper presented at the Third Research Seminar, ISME Commission on Music Therapy and Music in Special Education, Tallin, Estonia, USSR.

Taylor, D. B. (1991). *The biomedical theory of music therapy: A basis for our unique domain.* Founding Model Address presented at the annual meeting of the National Association for Music Therapy, San Diego.

Thaut, M., Brown, S., Benjamin, J., & Cooke, J. (1994). *Rhythmic facilitation of movement sequencing: Effects on spatio-temporal control and sensory modality dependence* [Abstract]. Fifth International MusicMedicine Symposium. International Society for Music in Medicine, San Antonio, TX.

Waldon, E. G. (2001). The effects of group music therapy on mood states and cohesiveness in adult oncology patients. *Journal of Music Therapy, 38,* 212–238.

Weber, S., Nuessler, V., & Wilmanns, W. (1997). A pilot study on the influence of receptive music listening on cancer patients during chemotherapy. *International Journal of Arts Medicine, 5*(2), 27–35.

Whipple, J. (2000). The effect of parent training in music and multimodal stimulation on parent-neonate interactions in the neonatal intensive care unit. *Journal of Music Therapy, 37,* 250–268.

Wilson, F. R. (1985). Music education for the handicapped: A keynote address to the Fourth International Symposium. *MEH Bulletin, 1,* 9–13.

Wilson, F. R. (1988). Music and medicine: An old liaison, a new agenda. *Psychomusicology, 7,* 139–146.

Wilson, F. R. (1989). The biology of music. In M. Lee (Ed.), *Rehabilitation, music and human well-being* (pp. 31–36), St. Louis, MO: MMB Music.

Woodward, S. C. (1992). *The transmission of music into the human uterus and the response to music of the human fetus and neonate.* Unpublished doctoral dissertation, University of Cape Town, South Africa.

Recommended Additional Readings

Harvey, A. W. (1992). On developing a program in music medicine: A neurophysiological basis for music as therapy. In R. Spintge & R. Droh (Eds.), *MusicMedicine* (pp. 71–79), St. Louis, MO: MMB Music.

Rudenberg, M. T., & Royka, A. M. (1989). Promoting psychosocial adjustment in pediatric burn patients through music therapy and child life therapy. *Music Therapy Perspectives, 7,* 40–43.

Schuster, B. L. (1985). The effect of music listening on blood pressure fluctuations in adult hemodialysis patients. *Journal of Music Therapy, 22,* 146–153.

Taylor, D. B. (1988). Therapeutic musicians or musical physicians: The future is at stake. *Music Therapy Perspectives, 5,* 86–93.

Taylor, D. B. (1997). *Biomedical foundations of music as therapy.* St. Louis, MO: MMB Music.

Thaut, M., Schleiffers, S., & Davis, W. (1991). Analysis of EMG activity in biceps and triceps muscle in an upper extremity gross motor task under the influence of auditory rhythm. *Journal of Music Therapy, 28,* 64–88.